Please feel free to order
additional copies at:

hepcman.com

Printed copies or ebooks are
available at this site.

Thank you!

Steve Chandler

Hepatitis-C and the working man

How I survived Interferon treatment

Steve Chandler

There are any number of people who have

influenced me in one way or another,

leading ultimately to this book. However,

the most consistent pats on the back and

boots in the butt belong to my mom...Thank

you mom, this one's for you.

Steve Chandler

January 2010

Let me start this with a warning, maybe a few warnings. I've had a checkered and interesting past. That's part and parcel of where I am today, so some of that has to come out to keep things in perspective. Some of it may be offensive or beyond understanding for you, but it's why I'm at this point and needs to be mentioned so it all makes sense. If I offend, please accept my apologies in advance.

I wrote most of this while under treatment. That may not be significant to you, but if you're going through treatment you'll see some things you may recognize. For those of you that haven't started treatment yet, in this I can recognize parts I wrote depressed, irritated, pissed off or on a fairly even keel. I don't want to scare you about the treatment, but I think you'll benefit seeing the treatment from one person's perspective. When your medical staff talks to you about the side effects, don't think "That won't happen to me" until you're in the treatment regimen. I thought the same thing until some of the side effects came to live with me for six months. My treatment didn't impact me as much as some, and was worse than some, which you'll find is a common theme. I'm writing this from my perspective only, in the hopes it helps you get though your treatment successfully.

You may feel like the Lone Ranger in this, like it's a disease only a chosen few get to experience for all the wrong reasons. A book I read regarding HepC and natural cures threw out a fact that really gave me some insight in this regard, along with conversations with my regular doctor. My doctor told me when I'd been infected for years with no side effects that it's estimated over 25% of the people with HepC had it and died of natural or other causes before it was apparent they had the disease. The book estimated that in addition to the one million diagnosed cases in the U.S. alone, there are over 5 million undiagnosed cases walking around out there. On a global level, that number jumps to *500 million* estimated cases. This disease crosses barriers of race, geographic location, age and social status seemingly with no regard for those barriers.

First warning: Remember, I'm only a doctor in my own mind. I have no training beyond what I have gleaned off the Internet, some self-taught natural remedies and cures, and a belief that most of the things that go "wrong" in our bodies can also be fixed by our bodies. I have self-diagnosed and treated for most of my life. This isn't from a distrust of doctors or the medical profession in general, but the attitude of "Why see a doctor when I'm already mending myself?"

2

Granted, there are some diseases and maladies that seem to be incurable, but I feel these occur less often than we've been led to believe. My Hepatitis-C got to a point where it looked like my options were the establishment's treatment or a liver donor list, and I finally agreed to the treatment. It's still a question that hits me occasionally... "Could I have picked up where I left off with naturopathic treatments and avoided the treatment?". My nurse answers this with a resounding "No!", but the question still lives in the back of my mind.

Before we take off down that road, let me give you some history for that perspective we talked about.

I

I grew up in the country, outside of a little town called Ely, Nv. I used to say I grew up on a farm, but that's not really accurate. It was 10 fenced acres 10 dirt-road miles from the nearest facilities of any type. There was no phone, no commercial power for the first few years we were there, and if we wanted TV we'd have to mount a 200' antenna to catch the signal over the ridge we snuggled up against. Sounds primitive, but in my opinion it was the best damn way to grow up.

I learned animal husbandry, as we raised our own beef, pigs and sheep for slaughter, chicken for eggs and Friday night dinner, and a milk cow to keep 3-6 growing boys in whole milk. Our chores were similar to a farmer's, milking twice a day, feed and water at least twice a day for all the animals, all this done before and after school around homework and a limited social life.

The ante was raised when my folks divorced. My mom kept the place with myself, a brother and a foster brother. Since Mom was keeping the financial wolves at bay, us boys learned independence and responsibility early and quick. Minor cuts and bruises, anything that wasn't gushing, wasn't worth worrying about…we learned to treat most of our injuries with a judicious amount of clean water and Corona bag balm. One of my clearest early memories was when our mare got her colt tangled up in a barbed wire fence as they were running alongside it. I can clearly remember boys holding legs and his head while my mom loaded the cuts with Corona and sewed him shut with a denim needle and heavy waxed thread. Say what you want, but we didn't have a vet bill, and less than a year later you had to know where to look to find any scars on that horse.

Having no TV, my interest in reading went from active to voracious. My brother was 4 years ahead of me, and when I'd read almost everything in the house I started borrowing his high school literature book to read short stories of authors I hadn't been exposed to by my grade school studies. This addiction has stayed with me since, which I've always been grateful for.

Six weeks after graduating high school I was headed for San Diego, CA for Navy Boot Camp. In high school I'd learned how much I liked alcohol, but didn't really have a clue the path I was starting down.

In the Navy I learned how to take drinking to a whole new level. I always excelled, and here was where I learned how to hide things. While growing up we ignored physical things that didn't seem a priority, and usually the rash or swelling went away by itself. Once I started really partying and having to perform a job also, I quickly learned how to hide whatever was bothering me, whether it was an oncoming cold or a killer hangover.

This seems a roundabout way to get to HepC treatment, but trust me, it all applies.

II

While in the Navy, I experimented with some illicit drugs. Grass never turned me on, all I did was laugh, eat and sleep. If I was going to do something illegal, I wanted to pack three days into 12 hours, I wanted to run at mach 10.

After I was discharged, I continued my drug usage. Somewhere in there someone introduced me to a much more efficient way to do speed. If you snorted it, it seemed too much stayed in your nose. Smoking it wasn't the rage then, but if you wanted more bang for your buck and didn't mind needles, shooting it was the way to go.

If you haven't gone down this road before, please don't feel the need to do it now. When you're speeding, and you've been on a runner with no sleep for a couple or three days, your priorities and limitations change dramatically. At that point, using a needle after someone else really doesn't matter, it's the drugs that are important.

I'm telling you this from my perspective then, 20 years ago. Somewhere in there I believe I contacted Hepatitis-C. It shames me, but I honestly

7

can't say that for sure, that's just the most reasonable timeframe.

While in the Navy, me and my budsters gave plasma regularly. Not out of the goodness of our hearts, not to benefit our fellow man, but for money! Get four guys together that are E-1's and -2's, broke, give them $10-15 apiece to lay on a bed for 90 minutes with a needle in their arm, and those boys have an almost instant party. After I got out of the Navy and moved to the Puget Sound area, things were pretty tight for my young family. By this time I had a wife, daughter and twin boys, with another son from a previous marriage that didn't live with us. Anyway, I went down and gave plasma again, this time for gas money and a little drinking.

They took my plasma the first time and told me my fluids would be screened before I could "donate" again. The next time I went to get drained, instead of being shown to a bed, one of the "doctors" took me into an office and told me my results showed I "may" have HepC. I think they have some liability to tell their donors, but they also can't tell you that yes, you have this disease. The doctor advised me this was a "double-blind" test, so he couldn't say

8

conclusively I had anything, but he had to advise me of the results and couldn't accept any of my plasma. I know this sounds like the clinic was wishy-washy (they were), but this was the early '90s, HIV and Hep strains other than A, things like that weren't as prevalent (or maybe were just kept more discreet).

Keep in mind, this was *years* ago. Since the clinic gave me such a convenient out and no one else had ever mentioned this disease, I thought their "double-blind" test must've been wrong (the doc said it might be, right?). At the time I didn't have a regular doctor, since even though I'd been away from the quasi-farm for around 10 years, I still didn't really need any more doctoring than I'd gotten with my Navy annual physicals. Since I knew nothing about HepC and "probably didn't have it anyway", I didn't tell my fairly new bride. Convinced I didn't have anything, it seemed easiest to let sleeping dogs lie. Yes, my outlook has changed drastically on these matters since then, thank you!

———————————————

So I knew there was a possibility I had HepC since the early '90s. I showed no symptoms, so it was an easy thing to just forget about. I did just that until 2003, when I started getting annual physicals.

There's enough cancer in my family that I wanted all the warning I could get, and knew from my reading habit that men were a target after 40. In 2004 I saw the doctor that had been my next ex-wife's (different wife than the 90's) GP during her pregnancy. When I told him it had been 12 years since my last physical (almost since I'd seen a doctor at all!), he ordered a full blood screening also.

I had changed my outlook on gifts that kept on giving by then. When he confirmed I had HepC antibodies in my blood, we moved forward with a liver biopsy to verify how much damage had been done and what our game plan should be from that point.

By this time I was single again, seeing a lady pretty regularly. Not to brag, hope I don't offend, but the sex was incredible. I agonized over it for a few days and let her know what my tests had turned up. If this disease could be transmitted by sharing wholesale amounts of most body fluids very regularly, she would have it also. She was due a physical fairly soon, and had her doctor check for hepatitis. She came back negative, good lord was I ever relieved!

This lady I've known and been a friend of since the mid '90s. We didn't become more than friends before 2004, but even as friends we were closer than a lot of married couples. After I told her about my diagnosis and had my meltdown, we talked about what steps I wanted to take next.

The biggie was the liver biopsy. Holy smoke that was unpleasant, even coasting on the Valium or whatever they give you to relax. This was in early 2005, and my understanding is it's done quite different now, but then it was one of the worst experiences I'd had and walked away from the same day.

The results came back better than I expected; there was minimal scarring on my liver, and with the levels in my blood my doctor recommended I attend an indoctrination for the interferon treatment that had pretty good success with the C strain.

In his opinion it would be good for me to explore my options, but I didn't have to act on them immediately. He said the levels in my blood didn't indicate the disease was active, so we had some time to work with as long as I continued to be tested.

I went to the indoctrination he suggested, and did my own internet education on natural cures. I also looked into the benefits, success and drawbacks to interferon shots and Ribavirin tablets that I'd be on for 6-12 months.

Okay, time for a little virology background. Several years after being diagnosed for sure, I learned that person to person transmission of this virus is rare via sex, estimated at less than 2%. Typically it's been through transference of blood, particularly with shared needles and blood transfusions until the early 90's. After that needles were still a major transmitter, but blood supplies began being routinely tested for HepC. Disturbingly enough, it's theorized HCV can possibly be transmitted via mosquito bites, like malaria and West Nile virus.

One other aside is sources of blood. I've always preferred my own towel, and have never shared things like toothbrushes. If you do, please pay attention! Many comparisons are drawn between the HepC (HCV) virus and the HIV virus. Not to minimize it, but currently HIV has infected an estimated 33 million people worldwide. By comparison, the HCV virus is carried by an estimated *500 million* people worldwide today. One reason for this difference is the survivability of each virus.

While HIV survives relatively short times absent the host, HCV virus has been found still active and infectious in dried blood samples *90 days old.* All that info leads to this...razors, toothbrushes, towels, washcloths, none of those should be shared while infected.

Okay, some more background for perspective. I was in major auto accidents in late 1999 and in 2000, 10 months apart. I was driving in both, was belted in both times, and judging by the cars shouldn't have survived either one. As much as I drank, I was stone sober in both wrecks and not at fault. The first one I lost my spleen, just bumps and bruises from the second one. However, being belted in, my hips and left shoulder took a pretty thorough beating twice.

The same doctor that did my physical after turning 40 had prescribed Vicodin for body aches. He would prescribe 30 tablets per scrip, and they would usually last me a year or more. That's indicative of my use of drugs. If I was stiff or sore, aspirin usually took care of it, or a good nights sleep. I was still in the "Steve, heal thyself" mode, and had no interest in prescription or any other drugs. That's where my head was at when I originally checked out the interferon and Ribavirin treatment for HepC.

Of course, my doctor told me I had to stop drinking when my blood work came back. I idled back some for a little while, but was soon right at the alcoholic level I'd been at before.

Here's another disclaimer! Remember, I'm only a doctor in my own mind. The treatments discussed in this book, other than the Interferon regimen, are what made sense to me. If they don't make sense to you, don't try them without investigating enough to put yourself at ease. I'm not making any statement as to the effectiveness of any cure I've tried, I just know they made sense to me. Let's be realistic, a large portion of something being effective is the patients belief in the treatment.

I had found two naturopathic cures that seemed logical to me. One was colloidal silver, which is a great antibacterial. It didn't occur to me that an antibacterial probably wouldn't have much effect on a virus. The other, hydrogen peroxide, oxygenates the body, and higher oxygen levels kill foreign bodies and boost your immune system from what I understand. I also regularly used dandelion root tea and tablets, and some liver-supporting natural supplements. I kept up this regimen for a couple of years, and my tests always came back with the antibodies present but no active HepC. Now human beings are a strange lot, or maybe it's just me. When you're doing something that is having benefits, why do you stop it?

Like I said, maybe it's just me, but after keeping a naturopathic regimen for a couple of years and having stable blood counts, I stopped treating it. It wasn't a conscious decision, it just got to be a hassle, I got lazy, the moon wasn't full, pick your favorite excuse or make one up for me. Keep in mind, though, I still had HepC, it's just that the counts were stable and I assumed that meant there wasn't further damage to my liver.

Anyway, about this time I lost my medical benefits, so I also quit getting my annual physicals. For a few years I lived and partied like I was still in my 20's, and when I got benefits I went to see my trusty doc after a 2-year hiatus. One of the concerns I had by this time was swelling joints. My blood work came back with elevated levels, high enough that he was concerned. He strongly recommended I take another look at the interferon treatment, even made me an appointment with the gastroenterology department.

So there I was. Anything that wasn't homeopathic or naturopathic was the devil, and I was

15

going to talk to the distributors of this poison. It went against everything in me, but after talking with the specialist, I took another hard look at this treatment.

I don't know if the natural course was keeping the HepC at bay or if it had just decided it was time to get on with the program, but my options were a lot more limited this time. I could restart the natural regimen I had been using and hope, I could get another liver biopsy to see what damage had been done so far and make a decision from there, I could say screw the biopsy and just start the interferon treatment, or I could ignore it and think about liver donor lists.

Holy smoke, there really wasn't much choice in my mind.

Restarting the natural regimen was possible, but I didn't know how effective it had been to start with, and the natural regimen was only supposed to keep it at bay, not kill it. My understanding was the interferon would actually kill the virus.

After my first biopsy I never wanted another, and another didn't make any sense to me. We knew when the HepC was inactive my liver had minimal

16

scarring, we knew the HepC had gotten active, and we knew when it gets active it attacks the liver, so we knew the results wouldn't be better than in 2005. Given the levels, there was a good chance the damage would now be worse, and if it wasn't it was just a matter of time.

So a biopsy was out, the natural route questionable, ignoring it wasn't even a viable option, so that left starting the treatment.

III

I know I'm repeating myself, but this treatment goes against everything I believe in when it comes to healing and medicine. This was a huge hurdle for me to get past, and the only comfort I could find was that it was for six months, and after that the virus would be gone forever. However, I still had to convince myself that six months of poison was worth it.

When I was originally diagnosed with this, it was a shameful thing for me. In the era and area I grew up in, STD's and lice and addictions were something hidden from the public eye. I still can't get used to lice treatment commercials on TV, in my mind it's something that you contact through general filth and a lack of personal hygiene, then you hide it, treat discreetly and immediately and never admit to. HepC is on the same level in my mind, but I had to let a few folks in on the news. There were some folks that needed to know regardless of the path I took, like the lady I was with and my kids (an edited version). Hiding it from them would be like being diagnosed with terminal cancer and not telling anyone, not something I could do. I felt my employer needed to know, especially if I started treatment, but also if I didn't and my performance started deteriorating.

This is kind of confusing, but since I had two instances where I was diagnosed and recommended treatment, there were two different sets of responses by me. The first time, I talked with my boss while I was weighing whether to start treatment or not. I found out his sister and husband had gone through the treatment. From his descriptions it sounded like they were lucky to have lived through the treatment. As I checked into this more it seemed to be a common theme; on this treatment you were lucky to be able to hold a job, it was basically like having the flu for 6 months given the added bonus of possible eye damage, diarrhea, nausea, body aches, insomnia, the list just went on! These side effects and my aversion to prescription medicine convinced me I didn't need to succumb to the treatment when I was originally diagnosed.

When I found out the levels were up and the disease active a few years later, deciding on the treatment was pretty simple. If six months of treatment meant never having to worry about HepC and donor lists again, I was willing to get it going.

IV

I have to say, my doctor and his nurses are the best. Here's a note you need to underline, highlight and tattoo backwards on your forehead...*You need to like your doctor and his nurses!* The treatment isn't dependent on this relationship (or maybe it is), but if I hadn't had two nurses I could call anytime and say I felt like reheated shit and had started gagging when I took my pills and reach an understanding ear, I don't know if I would have made it through the treatment. The staff I worked with weren't interested in bullshitting me or displaying everything in the best light, they were interested in me being informed and aware. When I ran into strange body functions, aches, reactions, or just plain wanted to quit breathing to make it all stop, they had already prepared me for it.

Dr. S. looked over my blood results and spent about 30 minutes with me going over pros and cons to the treatment. He didn't push the treatment, but I saw the writing on the wall all by myself; with this disease getting active, I could be less than a year from real problems that could be incapacitating or fatal. After speaking with him and Pam, one of his nurses, I decided to move ahead.

Pam did a phone interview with me a few days later. During this I was advised they wouldn't treat me if I was still drinking. Actually, Pam kept returning to the line "You really have to stop drinking.", until the last time I told her in a raised voice "OK, mom, last night was my last night!" That made the night before my last day as a drinker for at least the duration of the treatment. Three weeks later, after being dry for 23 days and having my eyes given the okay for the treatment, we met up at the clinic to do my first injection and go over side effects in detail.

A few days before my first injection is when the foundation between me and my medical staff was established. Pam called to set up an appointment for me to give some blood and a stool sample, the last things I had to do before starting treatment. She explained the blood helped set a baseline to evaluate my progress, and the stool sample was for tests they couldn't do with my blood. The blood I was fine with, who cares, but the stool? Pam told me "No worries, I think it's a diaper-type material, get a sample into that and seal it in a sample bag and bring it back. The sample just goes into a large sealed container." Well, that seemed straightforward enough, so I went by the clinic one morning and had blood taken, then told the lab tech I needed a stool sample kit also.

Here's where the fun starts! For those of you who've never done a stool sample, I was handed not a "diaper-like" material but a capped plastic cup about eight ounces in size. The instructions were the real capper, though.

"Your sample can't be contaminated (?) by anything, so the sample has to go directly in the cup, not out of toilet water or transferred by paper." *What?* First off, I thought the damn sample was nothing *but* contaminated by the time it was exiting, wasn't the whole idea behind evacuating it was getting rid of the junk etc that your body couldn't use? And second, straight into the cup?

I took the sample kit with grace, not even hinting to the lab tech the turmoil that was simmering under the surface. My mind was in high gear walking out, thinking around how the hell I was going to pull this off without needing a full-on decontamination after I was done. I could just see me in our nice bathroom, splatters of feces all over the walls and streaked on me with a pristine empty sample cup and bowel.

Wow, if that visual was a bit much I'm sorry, but in retrospect, well, it's funny as hell to me! Suffice to say I got the sample as ordered without mishap and returned to the clinic.

After dropping it off I walked over to the GI appointment desk and asked the receptionist if Pam was in. She was, but with a patient, so I left a note for her.

"Pam,

You owe me BIG TIME! Your stupid sample is in the lab, but "oh it's easy?" and "the big cup"? More like the size of a thimble, and it couldn't touch anything on its way to the cup, not even water! This bill WILL come due!"

Here's where the foundation comes in. I was amused by the whole thing, and signed the note with a smiley and my name. Several hours later I got a call from Pam just laughing her ass off. She thanked me for the sample and all I had to go through for it, and it took any bad right off the whole experience. Since then Jessica, the receptionist, has always known me by my first name, and my nurses always have a smile and hug for me.

Once I was sure my nurses could handle my sense of humor I got to have fun. Before my first shot appointment, I went to my favorite micro-brewery and bought a shirt for the occasion.

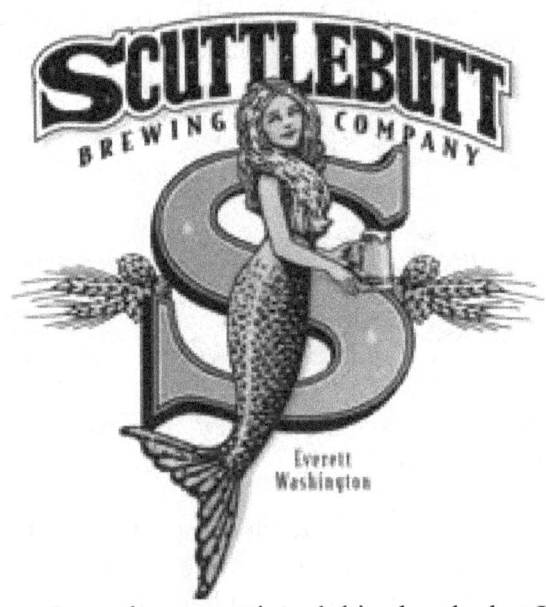

I may have mentioned this already, but I live in God's country for microbrews. One of my favorite places to eat and get a cold frosty beverage is Scuttlebutt Brewery. It's primarily a family-run business, great food and fresh brews on tap, in 6-packs, kegs, et cetera. They have some great shirts also, one that I bought specifically for "the day". On the front is a Scuttlebutt logo, and on the back is the quote especially for my doctor and nurses…

"The Liver is Evil…

It Must be Punished"

V

Oh joy! Let me give you a little more background first. My friend, coach, partner, room mate, whatever we are today, is also my support during this treatment. Here's another forehead tattoo for you...*You have to have a great support network for this to work!* She was there for my biopsy, there for the first indoctrination, and has been my crutch for these six months. My kids and ex's played a role in this also, being supportive and accommodating during the treatment.

I make these blanket statements but this book is like a supermarket; take what makes sense to you. All I know is these blanket statements were *critical* to my treatment.

One of her favorite accusations is calling me Superman. It's because of that mindset we talked about, where no one knows if I'm suffering or miserable unless I choose to let them know. I'm not encouraging you to become a sniveling wimp during this treatment, but the Superman syndrome won't serve you well, and could even hurt you.

The day I took my first injection was an eye-opener for both of us. I took the day off work, and had my shot about 1PM. In itself that was nothing to an ex-needle user, but about 4 hours later I went from okay to invalid in about 45 minutes. I had the chills and a raging fever, joint aches, stuffed dizzy head, the whole damn shooting match.

Both of my nurses told me ahead of time there was no problem with stopping the treatment if it got to be too much. However, that Superman syndrome goes beyond physical, and if there's a program that's been started, will benefit me to finish and is temporary, once I've taken the first step I'm on the path for the duration. So that's where my mindset was on the first day.

Each time I had an appointment I filled out a questionnaire that helped my staff track differences that won't ever show up in blood work and stool samples. On the next page you'll see my first one, what I look at now as a cocky, self sure form filled out by someone who has no flipping idea what he's signing up for. Of course, that's hindsight, and even that hindsight wouldn't change the course I chose.

Since your last visit, have you had any of the following? /16

☐ Chest pain	☐ Rash	☐ Heartburn
☐ Shortness of breath	☐ Vision changes	☐ Nausea
☐ Dizziness	☐ Mood changes	☐ Vomiting
☐ Cough	☐ New medical condition	☐ Appetite changes
☐ Fatigue	☐ Pain issues	☐ Weight loss/gain
☐ Fever	☐ Sleep problems	

Explain:

Since your last visit please rate the following:

Current energy level:	0 1 2 3 4 5 6 7 8 9 **10**	(0 = Bed bound -- 10 = Normal)
Irritability	0 1 **2** 3 4 5 6 7 8 9 10	(0 = None at all -- 10 = Extreme)
Anger	**0** 1 2 3 4 5 6 7 8 9 10	(0 = None at all -- 10 = Extreme)
Depression	**0** 1 2 3 4 5 6 7 8 9 10	(0 =None at all -- 10 = Extreme)
Thoughts of self-injury	**0** 1 2 3 4 5 6 7 8 9 10	(0 = Never -- 10 = Constantly)
Thoughts of harming others	**0** 1 2 3 4 5 6 7 8 9 10	(0 = Never -- 10 = Constantly)
Family/Social support	0 1 2 3 4 5 6 7 8 9 **10**	(0 = No support -- 10 = Excellent support)
Work status: ☒ Working	☐ Not working	☐ Retired ☐ Work restriction ___

Patient concerns or questions: None

1.
2.
3.

*********************************For clinic use only below this line*********************************

As you can see here, I had none of the issues in the first section and great numbers in the second section, with no patient concerns. This was filled out accurately and truthfully at the time.

For all the abuse and experience my body had in its forty-four years of mileage, I had nothing to complain about. Body aches and strange developments weren't anything aging wouldn't

28

explain, and I know I'm healthier and more fit than a lot of folks out there. Not blowing my horn, but being at this level starting treatment will make a difference later on, as you'll see.

Honestly, I feel much of my good health and acceptable 'wear and tear' on the gear (my body) is due to attitude. You'll see how that figures in on the next sheet I filled out.

Not everyone reacts to the treatment the same. For myself, nausea and irritability seem to be fairly consistent. They were there all the time, sometimes not so much, sometimes almost more than I could handle. Please don't see this book as the gospel according to Steve, it just aint so. I seem to have had the major symptoms, maybe some of the minor ones I ignored, but I was fortunate enough to be able to hold a job through the treatment and have a reasonably normal life.

We planned the first shot for a Friday on a weekend I didn't have any visiting kids. We wanted it to be low key and quiet for that first dose, so I could really critique the side effects without any distractions if possible. Our schedule was subject to the clinic, so I actually ended up getting my first dose on Thursday. Some of this I'm to blame for, since once I decided on the treatment it was push the envelope, full speed ahead let's get this started. Anyway, after my reaction on Thursday, I still ended up working on Friday (Superman, remember?). Or I showed up, anyway. Luckily, it was what I used to consider a light day, and I didn't work past eight that night.

I recuperated over the weekend, and just kept a close watch on my reaction to the injection and pills. The injection is once per week, the pills are two twice a day. It was recommended to me to do the injection around the same time of the same day each week, and to take the pills about 12 hours apart.

Now, being the genius I am, when my nurse told me it was a pill twice daily, I took one pill twice daily for the first 3 ½ days of my treatment. Then I got around to reading the bottle and realized I'd been on half doses since I'd started!

I immediately faxed a letter to my nurses so they'd be aware that the blood they would be getting the next day was after half doses.

This is a situation where having a good relationship with your medical staff is critical. Since I wanted to start this with all my cards on the table I faxed this list to them before treatment:

Attn: Pam B

Pam,

This is the routine stuff I do that may have an impact on the Pegasys treatment. I'm sending this to you now so you have a minute to look it over before our Thursday appointment.

Roasted Dandelion Root Tea	*1-3 20 oz. cups/day*
Green Tea	*2-3 20 oz. cups/day*
Coffee	*2-3 20 oz. cups/day*
Cod Liver Oil w/A & D supplement	*1/day*
B50 B-complex	*2/day*
Milk Thistle 500mg	*3/day*
E 400 I.U.	*1-2/day*
MultiVitamin & Mineral Supplement	*1/day*
Colloidal Silver	*varies*

Food-grade 35% Hydrogen Peroxide
varies (12 drops/8 oz. filtered water)

Vicodin 500mg   *2-3/month as needed*

Muscle relaxer   *<1/month as needed*

Tobacco (chew, 1 ½ cans/week)

Walk, avg. 2 miles @ 4mph
30 minutes, 3-5/week

See you Thursday!

Steve Chandler

As you can see, I was still with some of the naturopathic treatments to support my liver. This is just an example of the communication I personally recommend you have with your medical staff. I know I felt better knowing the staff was aware of what I was putting into my body during treatment, and honestly feel they appreciated being advised also.

They recommended I stop some for the duration, and gave others the green light. If I screw up my meds somehow, I can fax them in the middle of the night and by nine the next morning I've gotten a call to discuss it or just to tell me not to worry about it. What I'm harping on here is communication with your staff. These ladies may work for a local clinic, but for the duration of my treatment, they're *my* nurses, no one else's. What this has fostered and developed is completely open communication between us in both directions. Pam repeatedly telling me I had to stop drinking. Telling Kathleen I wanted to move my shot to a Thursday one week for convenience and being shot down. All your cards have to be on the table, baby, and you have to be able to *trust* your staff with that information. If you do the ganja, tell them. If you're ashamed but think you may have HIV, tell them. If you're fortunate enough to get someone you can talk to and cry with, it'll make your treatment much easier to accept.

VI

Okay, let's talk about your meds. The interferon shot was once every week for me, and the Ribavirin pills were twice daily. Since I work Monday – Friday, I decided Friday night would be pincushion time. After my reaction to the first shot, I also took my nurse's advice to "pre-medicate". With my aversion to drugs, I didn't pre-medicate for the first shot. After that experience I'm a solid gold believer in pre-medicating.

I have a pretty high tolerance for pain killers. Another disclaimer, did you hear it coming? Without consulting your doctor or nurses, **I don't recommend you take any dosage of anything.** That being said, on my shot nights I would take my pills like normal, then an hour later take a muscle relaxer and a Vicodin. An hour after that I'd do the shot, and usually stayed up about an hour after that and called it a night. With the chemical soup in me, I usually slept okay for about 6 hours, and if the house was quiet could sometimes sleep light for another couple of hours. This resulted in me sleeping heavy through most of the side effects. If you're still working up to the first shot and your staff recommends you pre-medicate please listen to them, gag Superman and *do it!*

My pills at night ended up being milk thistle (a liver-supporting herb), two PM Tylenol and two Benadryl along with the Ribavirin. In the morning it was milk thistle, fish oil, vitamin B multi-vitamin, green tea supplements. I'd hold off on the Tylenol in the morning and take a couple later in the day if things weren't sitting right. The Tylenol PM was for body aches, the Benadryl to assist sleeping. Yes, the Ribavirin messed with my sleep. I'm normally in bed awake at least 10 seconds after I decide it's time to sleep, until I started the treatment. If you have the urge to go ahead with these dosages, please refer to the above disclaimer and *talk to your nurses **first!***

Since I'm usually home by seven in the evening and I'm leaving for work about seven, that was my magic hour. On the weekends I slacken up a bit. If I sleep until 9, big frigging deal, I take them when I get up and then again around seven that evening. One thing recommended to me was taking them just before or after some food, a full meal if possible. With my schedule and my job (working on well systems, usually in the pucker bush backwater) there have been a few times I've taken the Ribavirin on an empty or nearly empty stomach, and it's not pleasant. In addition, according to my nurses the drug tends to like stomach lining, so if you'd like to avoid ulcers or worse, have a snack at least.

My first week of treatment I almost don't count, since I was doing my own thing and half doses. However, once I started full doses, by the next shot I was showing some of the side effects I'd been warned about. Remember, if you're on this treatment for six months, some of these side effects are going to be your day-to-day existence for six months or more. As I've already mentioned, I didn't have the worst reaction to this treatment, yours may be better or worse, it may be both depending on the day. One of my catch phrases has become taking it day by day, and sometimes minute by minute.

VII

I had changed jobs between originally being diagnosed and starting the treatment. The boss I had during the treatment was also a huge factor in my treatment. I have worked for this man in many capacities over the last 17 years. During that time I've worked for his companies the majority of the time, as software developer, dispatcher, plumber, well technician, accounts payable and receivable, human resources, payroll, etc. It was fortunate I was working for him during this, since he knew the skills I brought to the table besides what I could do in the field.

When I started the treatment I warned him my physical capacities and stamina may be impacted. A couple of weeks later we (my partner and I), had dinner with a co-worker and his girlfriend. There they got the straight scoop instead of Superman's version of the treatment, and I think they told on me to the boss. All I know is my performance in the field had degraded significantly, and suddenly there was a spot for me in the office, taking care of dispatching, software development and other administrative chores that the owner already knew I was well versed in.

By the end of my first month, I had kind of developed a routine. I was listening to my body more, and if I needed a break then Superman just needed to get over it. Sometimes I actually laid down for an hour or so in the middle of the day when I was off. Working in the office, I was doing better just by virtue of not wearing myself out daily with manual labor.

After a month I had an appointment with my doctor and one of his nurses to discuss progress. By this time in my mind they were the infamous little-known punk band, Dr S. and the Gastro Girls. During this checkup, I found out my red blood count was down, which causes fatigue, shortness of breath, general malaise, you get the picture. At least now I knew why I'd turned into a lightweight in the field…"What do you mean, I need a breather after backfilling six feet of ditch? Did I put on panties this morning or what?". Yeah, that was the original reaction, but now it made sense.

Overall the first month wasn't too bad. Don't get me wrong, it had its moments. It was either my 2nd or 4th shot, 30 minutes after it I was laying on my bed shivering and half delirious telling my roommate I just needed "a couple of minutes" to get on top of it. Soon I passed out and woke up 10 hours later. With the Ribavirin, I got used to joints being stiff and sore, head and body aches, insomnia, nausea from hell, and the real payoff, diarrhea! The crazy thing that you're going to have to accept is that whatever side effects you have, you probably won't have them consistently. I'll go a few days with decent bowels, then have a 5-day spree of not wanting to be further than 10 feet from a toilet.

Here's another example that drives me nuts. I started using Zicam about 4 years ago. Each spring I have about a week that's hell on my sinuses, and I used Zicam once and was sold. My nurses gave me the broad statement that side effects could include flu symptoms, and they weren't kidding. About a week into the treatment my sinuses were permanently stuffed it seemed, so I started using Zicam to fight it off and was dosing a solid 3-4 times a day for three weeks or so. That made it tolerable, and then suddenly for no apparent reason my sinuses were fine. That lasted about 5 weeks, and starting into my third month, I don't understand why, I had to start doing the Zicam again, 2-4 times per day if I wanted to breathe through my nose. Weird, no rhyme or reason.

All that being said, my first appointment after being on the treatment a month showed real promise.

Although my red cells were low, they weren't low enough for concern, just monitoring. My white cells were alright, and the biggie was the HepC virus was not detected, down from ten million detected units just a month before. That was great news, and Dr S. was almost giddy. (Can a reserved, quiet Japanese man be giddy? I think so, in the right circumstances).

Of course, one of my first questions was if the treatment was six months regardless. I don't want you to have that bubble burst, so just remember that when you start the treatment, it's for the whole duration, even if your labs come back good, sorry.

VIII

I recommended you to lose the Superman routine if that's how you deal with things. Now I have to temper that statement.

My mom is a big believer in "All things in moderation". Well, if you're stuffing all your symptoms and charging ahead, I think you're in for a train wreck, my friend. However, all things in moderation and all that crap....

The symptoms I experienced I could have let incapacitate. After sitting through a movie it took awhile, sometimes overnight, for my hips and back to feel alright again. Most of the mornings I went to work I had enough excuses to stay home on. Most weekends I used for recuperating from the shot, the last week and life in general, spending a lot of time in good books on the couch or my bed. But life still went on. We still went to movies, I still taxied my kids around, I even officiated at a Saturday wedding for my niece in Montana one weekend! See, life goes on, and if you let Superman stuff your discomfort sometimes and just go for it, it'll make things move along just like they're supposed to.

I have to tell you about that wedding, and I'm telling you this not to beat my chest, but to give you hope.

Before I started my treatment, my niece in Montana asked me to officiate their wedding. Being a five-time divorcee, at first I thought they were joking, but they were dead serious. This was about two weeks before I started treatment, but the timing didn't matter, I'd have told them yes if I was on my deathbed.

After starting the treatment I wondered how well this would go, knowing how I felt sometimes on Saturday. I asked my nurse if I could move the shot to Thursday for one week and she recommended against it, so I was sticking with that schedule. Being in the Seattle area and both working, we took Friday off, picked up a rental car and headed east Thursday night.

Again with the Superman mindset. When I take a driving trip, there's point A and point B, everything in between is usually incidental. I don't usually take trips to sightsee, but because I have something at the end. So a 12-hour drive like this would usually be done in one shot with 3 stops for fuel, bathroom and a quick bite. Well, my roommate put the kibosh on that early on, insisting we stop roughly midway and get a hotel room, which was the best thing we could have done. We stopped in Spokane around 10, got a decent nights sleep and finished the trip Friday around midday.

I could have done it in one shot, had done it several times before. But because I was listening to my body and my support instead of my mindset and ego, it went much better. We kicked around Great Falls getting the tux fitted and helped with the setup Friday, begged off the drinking Friday night and returned to the hotel so I could dose up.

I pre-medicated a little heavier than normal and slept hard. The next day we helped with some more setup, did hair and makeup (my roommate did, anyway), and pulled off the wedding without a hitch. I was nervous, this being my first wedding on this side of the altar, and knew the stress could have physical side effects, so I wasn't shy about dosing during the day within reason.

Remember, this is from the drug anti-christ. I'm telling you this as an example – if you're going to live a normal life and want to pack a weekend with travel, visiting and stress, plan for it! Pre-medicate, rest, plan breaks or stops *and keep them*, and listen to

44

your body. It will tell you when it's getting pissed early enough for you to decide you can medicate or you need to stop.

Here's one interesting aside that might help you. When we were at that wedding, the day before, one of my daughters and I were verbally sparring like we always do. I made a comment about something holding me up, and she said something about the bar holding me up after a few hours.

My support lady heard this, and a little bit later took all my kids and my ex aside and defined for them what this treatment meant for me, and what changes it wrought in me, like the dry spell. Now understand, with my Superman complex, none of these people knew I'd been dry for a couple months by then. They also didn't realize that I had to take a shot that night, before the wedding, and maintain the next day. They also didn't realize that I was treating myself with lethal chemicals in the "hope" that the virus would die before I did. Just an aside, remember that if you're like me, not everyone realizes what you're going through. When you get deep into treatment, you may forget that and assume those around you know what's going on, but you may not have taken them into enough confidence for them to really know.

One of the biggies that I had to learn to deal with was irritability and depression. Usually I'm a very positive, upbeat individual, and my nurses warned me that may be put to the test under treatment.

The irritability was something that was sort of two-pronged. I could get irritated over a song, someone repeating a noise one too many times, pretty much anything by this point in treatment. To compound this, my skin became hyper-sensitive about this time. I'm a touch freak in all the right ways, love and need physical contact, even if it's just a finger rubbing the back of someone's hand. However, as symptoms progressed, my skin became so sensitive even clothes were torture spawned by demons sometimes. This went from irritation to physical pain during treatment.

Remember the first questionnaire I filled out? Even though I was dealing with the symptoms, comparing the questionnaires in January and March, there's a huge difference.

Date: 3-4-08
Tx Week: _Tuesday_ _legacy?_
Rx: _Rd 3 32_

Since your last visit, have you had any of the following?
- ☐ Chest pain
- ☒ Shortness of breath   H&H
- ☒ Dizziness
- ☐ Cough
- ☒ Fatigue
- ☒ Fever *chest*

- ☐ Rash
- ☐ Vision changes
- ☒ Mood changes
- ☐ New medical condition
- ☐ Pain issues
- ☒ Sleep problems

- ☐ Heartburn
- ☒ Nausea
- ☐ Vomiting·
- ☒ Appetite changes
- ☒ Weight loss/gain   *bowels*

Explain:
Lost 15-ish lbs, lighter appetite, a bit of insomnia due
fatigue/dizziness/shortness of breath - lost my stamina @ work

Since your last visit please rate the following:

Current energy level:	0 1 2 3 4 5 ⑥ 7 8 9 10	(0 = Bed bound – 10 = Normal)
Irritability	0 1 2 3 4 5 ⑥ 7 8 9 10	(0 = None at all – 10 = Extreme)
Anger	0 1 ② 3 4 5 6 7 8 9 10	(0 = None at all – 10 = Extreme)
Depression	0 1 2 ③ 4 5 6 7 8 9 10	(0 =None at all – 10 = Extreme)
Thoughts of self-injury	⓪ 1 2 3 4 5 6 7 8 9 10	(0 = Never – 10 = Constantly)
Thoughts of harming others	⓪ 1 2 3 4 5 6 7 8 9 10	(0 = Never – 10 = Constantly)
Family/Social support	0 1 2 3 4 5 6 7 8 9 ⑩	(0 = No support – 10 = Excellent support)
Work status: ☒ Working ☐ Not working ☐ Retired ☐ Work restriction ____

Patient concerns or questions:
1. _stopped brev – feels like that is reason behind wts_
2. _feels like he is just more awake-_
3. _has been using benadryl for sleep - not working_

****************For clinic use only below this line****************

_____
_____
_____
_____
_____
_____
_____

Recommendations:
1. _may need something for sleep -_
2. _____
3. _____

Helbec 0005

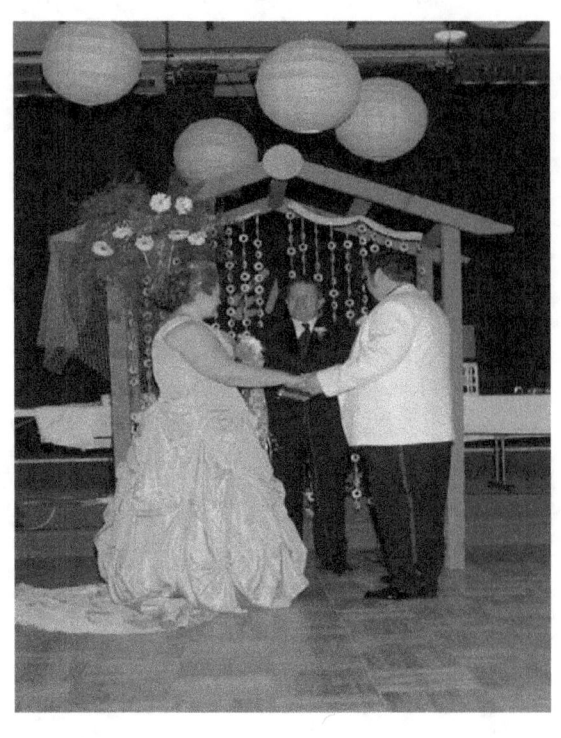

Yes, I really did marry them!

IX

My roommate has said for years that I may suffer from seasonal depression. She saw dark moods and drinking spike during the winter, and we had a couple of Christmas seasons that would have ruined most relationships. They weren't a joint effort, either, they were about 90% me. I haven't been a holiday person since I graduated high school, but this attitude had been magnified during the last few years and was hell recently. That changed this last holiday season, in which I had a pretty good time and accepted it as temporary and something necessary for my kids if nothing else. That sounds kinda blasé for the holidays, I'm sure some of you are saying, but it was the best I had dealt with a holiday season in years.

Anyway, a couple months later I filled out the questionnaire and started treatment. I mention the holidays so you understand I'd been through what was historically my worst time already that year, then started treatment in what should be my "better time". It wasn't planned that way, it just sorta happened, but in retrospect the timing was probably best.

The questionnaire specifically asked about thoughts of hurting yourself or others, and my nurses asked about the same things, the answers being an easy no. When I returned for a follow-up seven weeks later, the answers were still no. However, in the next two weeks something changed. The most frustrating thing about this was that, like the diarrhea, nausea, etc, there was no rhyme or reason that I could identify.

There were times before treatment that I drank, which was most of the time. And then there were times, looking back, that I was seeing which would break first; my body, my bank account, or the rum distilleries. During those times, the day after I would function with a huge black hole driven though my chest, not caring about or for anything, just wanting it all to end. Did I have thoughts of suicide? I'd be lying if I said no, but they weren't something I dwelled on, just something that would wave at me from the edge of my thoughts and then be dismissed. As the alcohol left my system and my mind started working clearly again, the thoughts and the hole would go away.

However, eight weeks into treatment, Friday and the wonderful shot came around. It was a rough week, no energy or appetite to speak of, which seemed to be more common as I progressed in the treatment. I noticed early on that by the time Friday came, I was beyond ready for the work week to be over, and the weekend recuperation became more critical as each week passed. This week I did my regular pills on schedule, did the shot, was up a couple of hours and hit the sack, just business as usual by this time. When I woke up Saturday there was just no drive, it felt like I'd drank heavy Friday and missed the regular hangover, but had the same emotions. While I didn't feel like I was in a danger zone, I certainly listened more to my body and emotions that weekend. Once again those thoughts were waving from the sidelines, so I concentrated on interacting with people, not on a deep emotional level but just on a social level to keep the mind and emotions positively engaged. When I hit this type of funk while drinking, thought had really been anesthetized for awhile, so I just let the mood take its course. However, seeing these symptoms while sober, I recognized I was better off going through the day to day motions and keeping my mind occupied rather than giving myself time to brood.

I don't know if Sigmund Freud would have approved of my self-treatment, but it worked. That's something I hope you see throughout this book, I didn't necessarily do exactly what was recommended, but what worked for me at that moment. Like I said, the most frustrating thing about your symptoms may be that they're not consistent. They didn't read the rule book before coming to visit you, and they're bastards with attitude. Sometimes you'll have to take what's been advised, bend it to fit where you're at right then, and go with it.

Irritability was another symptom of depression that I thought would pass me by. I'm rarely irritable, but when I am can usually undo it with a change of scenery or focus. That was true up until about my third week, when I realized one day on a job site that this specific thing about a co-worker and friend gave me the urge to just bust him in the chops. I've had my share of barroom and back alley tussles, but it's always been with cause or alcohol or both, never just because someone irritated me. This was the point when I realized that another wonderful side effect had come to roost and may stay with me for the next few months.

Let me just take this opportunity to say to all the ladies that read this book, I'm sorry. For over 40 years I've thought women must be psychotic to give in to the emotional swings, hormonal hell and irritability just because they were menstruating. Alright, I'm sorry, damnit! After being exposed to a little of what you must feel each month, I'm a bit more understanding now, and a lot more sympathetic.

The only thing different is I experienced it more on than off for six months solid, but all of you still get props from me if you have indoor plumbing.

The irritability did stick around, in fact. The language around our house is a lot like a combination sailors bar and truck stop sometimes, which we're alright with. With the irritability level on the rise, there were some very colorful exchanges. But again, I was focused on listening to my body and emotions during this time, and early on started recognizing the irritability coming on. Because of that, these exchanges had a humorous current when they could have turned into something ugly. I never purposely hurt anyone, physically or with words, even though it was tempting sometimes, to be honest. That's not who I am, just where I was at in the moment.

Sometimes it was enough to just get on my computer, listen to some tunes and play Spider Solitaire while I unwound. Other times nothing relaxed until I slept. A good action or comedy would turn the tide sometimes. I've been of the opinion for a long time that if you don't laugh every day, that day's wasted and you'll never get it back. Sometimes I just went to youtube and watched Jeff Dunham clips until I *couldn't* maintain the irritability. Sorry, if you can watch more than 5 minutes of Peanut and not lighten up, you may be past helping.

Another thing that helped was being alone. I know that works for some and wrecks others, but for me it was occasionally the best thing. There's some Mike Doughty lyrics that fit me perfectly at times:

"Slow down, don't fuck with my heart,

I want to be left alone here with my monsters."

The irritability sometimes acted like a stealth emotion also, as an added bonus. One day I was physically out of sorts all day, carried over from the night before. I maintained at work about half a day and had to call it, went home and took it easy and seemed to be a little more balanced. Then one little thing that normally would have mildly irritated me came along and before I had a chance to get a handle on it I was in a full-blown rage. This is from someone who needs a lot of help from plenty of alcohol to find that kind of emotion, and even then doesn't quite get to where he thinks he wants to go, however twisted that may be. The rage rose and I fortunately had to take a drive with one of my kids. I say fortunately because driving alone I may not have cared much, but having one of my kids riding shotgun I couldn't be the asshole I dearly wanted to be. Since I had to behave, the anger ebbed away, and by the time I got home again emotionally I was more balanced. I don't say better because I wasn't. The side effects didn't go away, but I'd had time to bring things back into control, to recognize the hair trigger that I was currently on, and to get a firmer grip on the emotions so I'd know whether to deal with the next thing or absent myself for a moment. You know, maybe I'd want to be left alone here with my monsters, and if that's what worked that time, alright.

X

Another development in the second month was with my eyes. (Good lord, I feel like I'm talking about my pregnancy with all the references to months and weeks, but I guess we gotta keep track somehow. Just know I'm full of shit if I say "In the last couple weeks my belly button popped out like the timer on a frigging turkey".) One of the requirements before starting treatment was an evaluation by an ophthalmologist to ensure my eyes would handle an interferon-based treatment.

About 18 months before I started treatment I had Lasik done, and hoped the follow up I'd had a year after my Lasik would suffice. If you're thinking the same thing let me prematurely pop that bubble for you too. Whatever tests and observations they make when checking your progress after Lasik doesn't give a doc the information he needs before starting you on an interferon-based regimen.

By being required to have this evaluation, I logically assumed the drug regimen may have side effects that could impact my eyes. In the second month I started noticing my eyes were a bit more sensitive to light. Right around the rollover from the second to third month, my eyes started to hurt. This was a pain like I'd never experienced before, an actual ache of the orb of my eyeball, like my eyeballs themselves had become too large for the socket.

Like the other symptoms, this wasn't consistent. I noticed it peak the first couple of times about 12-18 hours after my injection. In that timeframe, sunlight through a light overcast was enough to send me searching for sunglasses, and at its peak the world was too bright even through my ultra-dark, mirrored shades.

Again, there were different ways to deal with it. I'm sure you've noticed the inconsistencies with how I dealt with things on different occasions, and this challenge was no different.

After experiencing it the first time I could recognize the warning signs and take steps to handle it. When my eyes acted like they didn't want to rotate in their sockets, when I got a low grade ache behind my eyes, I knew it was times to take steps. The first thing was to close my eyes, especially if I was riding in a car. If I could keep my eyes from trying to track things sometimes that was enough, just to close my eyes for an hour or so. If I was home, a dim room helped, a nap if possible sometimes turned the tide in short order.

57

We've already talked about my reading habit. Whenever I left the house to go 30 minutes or more away, I'd take a book if I wasn't driving, and that didn't change when I entered treatment. However, when the symptoms started coming on, it was also time for the book to be shelved for awhile. Sometimes that was an hour, once it was more like a day plus.

Even when your eyelids are closed, your eyes move around some. When I'd "check out" for a little while, if the ache kept building it was time to find some aspirin. Once again, I have a high med tolerance, so know your own limits and discuss this with your treatment staff, and don't take my doses as a standard.

I'd start with aspirin, and if an hour didn't make a difference I'd usually take a Vicodin and depending on how things were developing, a muscle relaxer. This combination wasn't common, since it would land me on the couch or bed for at least a few hours, but if the eyes were bad enough and the timing was right (like I wasn't at work) that would be my final solution.

I'm sure I'll have some more information on this later. If it's a temporary side effect that stay's manageable I'll be quizzing the Girls about it, you can guarantee.

XI

Here's another side effect that I would have never expected; I had more *money*. What the hell?

I've always been a bit or a lot financially challenged. It seemed living paycheck to paycheck was my lot in life. But about six weeks after starting treatment, I started having money left in my account when payday rolled around.

Being the person I am, I just had to know what was going on. I started tracking things, and the only thing that had changed that would impact my finances was that I'd stopped drinking.

In talking with my roommate (who did Weight Watchers so was on top of points and calories etc), I realized I was consuming 2,000-3,000 liquid calories *per day*. That translates to most peoples total daily caloric intake. Don't do your calculations on light beer, or the phony beers out there. Not to name names, but nothing I drank was associated with big-hooved horses or Rocky Mountain spring water. Oh no, I feel like I live in the microbrew capital of the world, and my beers were heavy, usually between 7-12% alcohol and looked like a cross between black coffee and motor oil. My god, they were the best!

Well, the calorie count was high, and these brews aren't cheap. Once I translated the calories to ounce to number of bottles to price per bottle, I realized I had a $10-50 per day habit. Holy crap, no wonder my paychecks didn't seem to go very far! And that didn't even accommodate the 1-2 bottles of rum per week at $15-29 per bottle.

You might wonder "Why is he taking off on this side trip?". Well, for a substantial number of us out there, this isn't a side trip but a major part of the treatment. I could be totally wrong on this, and if I am accept my apologies.

I know that a drinking habit led me down paths I would have never chosen sober. If I track these paths logically, one major happening to the next, I have to wonder if I'd have HepC if I didn't have a drinking habit. Am I blaming alcohol? No, to lay blame all I have to find is a mirror, but laying blame isn't the point.

The point is, I think a majority of us treated ones were given the choice by our own set of Gastro Girls to either quit drinking or don't start the treatment, because a majority of us are hard drinkers or alcoholics. I don't have any facts or figures to back this up, this is just my gut feeling. If this

61

feeling is accurate then there's a few things I have to bring up.

First, if you were told to stop drinking, said you would, entered treatment and kept drinking, even at a lesser rate, you're fucking up. I wish there was a kinder way to put it, but the point has to be made and if a little constructive French drives the point home, there ya go.

The disease we've contacted eats your liver, you know that, right? The alcohol we pour down our gullet eats your liver slower, and you know that, right? The treatment you're starting or have started impacts your liver, and you know that, right? Well then, if you know all this, you're in treatment and still drinking, maybe you need to know this…*You're human! Your liver and other organs are only going to take so much abuse and then they're all shutting down on you. You've abused your liver voluntarily, possibly in the process contacted this disease, now you're willing to abuse your liver some more to cure the disease, **get a handle on it and stop drinking for six goddamn months!***

I would say thank you, I'm over it, but I'd be lying. I had to put it out there bluntly 'cause that's who I am. If that got through to you when nothing else would, you'll get no apologies from me. Remember earlier, talking about your medical staff, yes *your* medical staff, the folks you told your deepest secrets to so they could treat your HepC the best? I said then there has to be trust both ways, but you're betraying that trust if you're still drinking, and you're hamstringing your treatment. If this is the point you're at, in my opinion you have a simple choice to make: Stop drinking or stop the treatment.

When I told Pam I'd stop drinking, it sounds like a flippant, easy decision on my part. It was anything but easy, please believe me. If you have a drinking habit, you know it was not an easy statement to stick with, however I represented it. But I was focused and determined that once the treatment was my answer, I'd do whatever it took to make the treatment work. If giving my liver a break was required so I could temporarily abuse it with medicine, so be it. The end justified the means. If you end up making the same decision, I hope you stick with it for the duration; your treatment regimen, your body and your liver will all thank you.

If you're starting treatment or have already started and think "Well, an occasional drink won't hurt", I'll gladly pop that bubble for you right here and now and admit for you that yes, I'm human too.

On two occasions a smoking good microbrew was just too tasty to pass up. The first time, one beer (20 oz.) and a healthy shot of rum was good for about an hour. Then I started feeling like any misery I'd felt that far into the treatment was just a preview. My entire body ached, radiated heat, shivered, throbbed, I think you get the picture. I'd experienced some real discomfort up to that point in the treatment, but throw a little alcohol in on top of that to really take it to the next level.

Now why you'd experience that kind of a reaction and try the same experiment a few weeks later is beyond me, but I did, and the strange thing was, I got the same results! No fun folks, and the worst part about it was I'd volunteered for the treatment, said I wouldn't drink and then did anyway, so we could add guilt to the mix. I've never taken Anabuse, but have discussed it with people who have. If my reaction was any indicator, drinking on this treatment regimen could be compared to drinking on Anabuse.

My roommate has asked me if I'm going to be a wildman the day after treatment is over. I can't honestly answer that because I'm not there yet, but I can give you this:

I know the medications I've poured in for months won't leave my body the day I'm done with treatment. If I remember right, if you're capable of having kids, the recommendation is 6 months after treatment before you conceive a child to avoid birth defects. That part kinda went right past me since I'm fixed, but the idea is there's enough chemicals in your system to screw up a fetus half a year later, so I'm sure they'll react to drinking the same way six months after treatment as they did during treatment.

That being said, I'll be very careful about drinking for at least the first year after treatment. Will I drink again? I think I'd be kidding myself to say no, and I've kind of learned about saying never. However, after learning about the damage I've done to my liver with alcohol and disease, I can't justify being the drinker I was, and being an alcoholic, I think an occasional drink after treatment could easily turn into a habit again, and that's nowhere I want to be. So the long and short is, after treatment I'll be 6 months and three weeks dry…not a bad starting point to continue with.

As you drinkers know, it's one day at a time. I wish I could without doubt commit right now to never drinking again, but I'm not there yet. When I have treatment completed, get 3 months past that and have a drink that makes me want to find a coffin and crawl in, maybe that will be the time. For now, I'm focused on not drinking for the duration of treatment, and the future will keep its secrets.

XII

Okay, we have to back up a bit now to get you current, if that makes sense. If it doesn't, it might after you've read this.

As I've already said, I hate prescription medicines, or anything that isn't naturopathic and a proven herb or supplement. Finding myself in the position of feeling like a prescription drug czar for six months wore on me, I could say daily but it was actually more often than that. Sometimes I'd find myself spun up with the morning dose, spun up at the evening dose, and during the day suddenly realizing I was a goddamn Petri dish for chemical reactions that my body wasn't liking one bit.

Yes, I'm bitching, but I always came around to the realization that I didn't have it nearly as bad as some others who have done this treatment. It helped to be conscious of this, because even on my worst day, well, it could be even worse. Count your blessings and all that happy crap.

Anyway, after five weeks of treatment, I had a follow-up with Dr S and Kathleen. They were very happy with how I was reacting to the medication and the levels of HepC virus. My white and red blood-cell counts had shifted, the white to the good, the red towards the bad but not in any danger zone. When we discussed blood counts I remembered Kathleen five weeks before, when I took my first shot. At that time she advised me the several blood-draws through the six months were to first establish a baseline of pre-treatment and then monitor how my blood was reacting to treatment. She also told me that my interferon shot may not be the only one in play during those six months, depending on my blood numbers.

Count those blessings, baby. I could have ended up with at least two other weekly shots to stabilize the red and white blood counts if I had reacted differently. The reason I bring this up is a reminder for myself as well as information for you. The second questionnaire was filled out on my second office visit, and there were some differences, particularly in weight, insomnia and nausea. As I've already pointed out, the pre-treatment me was a little different. I was a sleeping machine when it was nighty-night, and can count on one hand the number of times I'm nauseated in a year.

After reminding myself that I was avoiding more shots by the blessing of good reaction, we discussed the changes. I knew from the first appointment that sometimes the thyroid lost its mind during treatment, luckily that wasn't my case. However, between the nausea and a reduced appetite from the chemicals, I'd dropped about 20 pounds by my second appointment. Now I didn't mind that one bit, but was keeping an eye on it to make sure it didn't get out of hand. Understand, in my opinion when I entered treatment I had an easy 40 pounds I could do without, so being halfway there didn't bother me as long as I was eating reasonably.

Let's talk about that a bit and then we'll discuss my "drug revelation". My appetite has always been pretty good, I can dust a steak and baker, wash it down with a couple cool frosty beverages and be set for the night, circa pre-treatment. Now I've heard that in American restaurants the portions are such that you can get your meal and a go-box, halve everything on your plate, eat it and take the other half home for lunch the next day and still maintain a 2,000-2,500 calories/day diet easily. I've also heard it's much healthier to eat several smaller meals than 3 big meals per day, but have never been able to break out of that "three squares per day" mentality. Well, introduce us to treatment!

When my appetite went to hell, I found that a big part of it was just the portion size. I was still hungry, just couldn't load up the plate like I was used to. Trust me, during the first few weeks I'd look back on what I'd had for dinner and hoped I could still cast a shadow the next morning.

With the smaller portions, I found myself packing a much different lunch. I'd usually pack two pieces of fruit, maybe a yogurt, some cheese sticks and either a big old sandwich or a couple pieces of chicken, something like that. Once treatment started kicking in, that didn't change radically, but it did fundamentally. Lunch now consisted of a sandwich, PB & J, smoked turkey & pepper jack, something like that, but not as thick and cut in half. I found sometimes eating just half was just right, but really had to *allow* myself to do that.

The real difference was in snacking. There were days the sandwich or chicken didn't get touched, just a piece of fruit and cheese stick mid-morning, same around midday, then a yogurt and a granola bar around mid-afternoon. By the time I got home from work, I'd have an appetite but not raging by any means. Usually some small portions, probably $1/3^{rd}$ of what I was used to, would keep me just fine.

Now remember, not only am I not a doctor, I aint a dietician either. Check with your staff, especially if you have a large weight loss or gain after starting treatment. I know that my diet drove my roommate (remember, Weight Watchers warrior, and she's done very well at it healthily) to distraction sometimes. She saw the weight loss, questioned me occasionally about actual poundage, but never called the Gastro Girls and told on me, so I guess it was within safety zones. One thing I didn't change much was the eating schedule I was on for breakfast and dinner. I've always loved breakfast anytime of the day, and with my 7AM/7PM Ribavirin schedule, I had to eat around that time whether I wanted to or not. Breakfast never really suffered, always a bowl of cereal or a couple scrambled eggs with last nights pork chop diced up in there, but there were times the best I could do for dinner was a cup of yogurt before taking my pills.

I've got to throw this line at you, used to use it on a guy at work that hates yogurt. Used to tell him as I finished a cup "MMM, yogurt! You know, of all the rotten dairy products, I'd have to say yogurt's the best!" Maybe it was that growing up on a farm and never being able to throw away leftovers, but that always cracked me up.

71

Okay, so much for dieting. As an aside, that diet change started in the first month, and pretty much has stuck since then. Remember from the little introduction, I started writing this in the third month, so this is all real time now. I don't see that diet changing much over the next few months, and it's not a bad habit to be in, in my opinion.

XIII

I was having a lot of trouble sleeping from the first week on. My Girls had told me to try a couple benadryls 30 minutes to an hour before bedtime, that would help. By the second appointment, that wasn't enough pretty regularly. Being Dr. Steve and Superman, I had to self-dose for awhile.

Now remember, I have a high tolerance for pain meds. After having a couple almost sleepless nights, I took a Vicodin with my PM meds and benadryl. That seemed to work pretty good, although some nights I'd add a muscle relaxer to the mix, just to be sure.

I looked back on this after a few weeks and thought "Bullshit!" Here I was, the king of no prescription drugs, dosing with narcotics nightly to help me sleep. When I had my second appointment, I marked on the sheet that insomnia was up, and told Kathleen how I was dealing with it. She was convinced I'd be better off with a sleeping pill, which I thought was total crap. I saw it as dumping another chemical into an already unacceptable mix.

Dr S. decided to give me a prescription for Ambien, but was very hesitant to issue it. I thought he wasn't going to, with his attitude, and secretly I was just fine with that, but he did. Kathleen also had him issue a prescription for irritability, which I never had filled.

I tell you that 'cause I'm human. My Girls told me some things, they could have just saved the air, I wasn't hearing it no matter how many times they repeated it. Kathleen and Pam, my Gastro Girls, hold a very special place in my heart, and I'm so appreciative of what they helped me though, but my mom holds a special place in my heart and I didn't do everything she said either. The mood enhancers or whatever they were was a case in point.

My doctor wrote the sleeping pills scrip, but cautioned me to start with ½ a pill *only when necessary*. Well, I don't know, at seven or eight when I can take the pill, if it was necessary that night, let it kick in around 9:30 or 10, I can still get eight-ish and be alright the next day. When I realized *it was necessary* because I'd read 75 pages and wasn't close to sleep and it was after midnight, I was afraid to take it and oversleep or be a zombie the next day. That was when I realized I had to find a balance.

By the fourth week I'd had them, I think I'd taken 3 sleeping pills, so 6 nights I used them. They worked pretty well, did what they needed to, and I didn't have to do the Vicodin or muscle relaxer. *That* was the balance I needed to find. Again, it was critiquing and listening to my body…was benadryl enough tonight, or do I cut the happy pill in half? There were evenings that I could feel the tired coming on, those nights benadryl and a good book would have me nodding by 10. Other nights I was spun up, couldn't unwind and sleep felt like the last thing I'd try. On those nights, it usually wasn't a good clean burn like you feel when the energy level is up and all the juices are doing what they're supposed to. No, those nights it was like waiting for a train wreck you knew was coming, all jangley and scatter-brained. Those nights I finally started submitting to the staff and doing what I needed to. It was giving in, but the benefits were tremendous. Early on I recognized if I slept badly the night before, the following day was probably going to be an imaginative version of hell. What pushed me over the edge with the sleeping pills was that I knew the price I'd pay the next day if I didn't get some decent sleep, and I knew that my best healing and body maintenance went on during that sleep.

If you experience the insomnia, listen to your medical staff and treat it just like you're treating your HepC. If sleeping pills are the devil to you, maybe a lighter dose or cut a pill in half. Before I gave in to that, I tried several naturopathic routes, valerian root and bedtime tea and a few others, but they never had any impact on sleeping during treatment. I've used those successfully before treatment, so I know they work, but not for me in this case.

So the short version is if you're dosing yourself with one chemical to avoid taking another, step back and take a look at what you're doing. In my case, it didn't make any sense to me to take one or two other narcotics to avoid a sleeping pill that was designed for what I needed.

Okay, 'nuff said on that, with one other "What the hell?" comment. During my first appointment and shot, Kathleen told me I had to be careful of my water intake for the entire treatment, as most of these drugs tend to dehydrate you. Her rule of thumb was if you didn't get up at least once each night to pee, you weren't drinking enough water. I'm telling you, when I finally got to sleep some nights and woke up two hours later to stumble into the bathroom, I was cursing my Gastro Girls the whole damn way.

XIV

Taking my 11th shot tonight, so I'm ten weeks into this. Up until now, it hasn't been a breeze by any means, but it's been manageable. This last two weeks I've started noticing some effects that seem to be more long-term and a little concerning.

My jobs have historically been with small companies. Usually benefits were not part of any package, or if they were it seemed prohibitively expensive, especially for Dr Superman (that's me). When I realized this treatment may be my only viable option, I had just re-established benefits. This was through a builders association statewide, and one of their rules were only full-time employees could have benefits.

Before I got benefits I was working 4-day weeks and using three-day weekends for my real estate business. However, when my real estate business was non-existent I decided to go to 40 hours per week. The owner had mentioned to me earlier that he'd get me on benefits if I'd like, but at the time I wasn't "full time". Once that changed, I got the benefits, set up my first physical in years, and you've already read where that got me.

My employer made some allowances for me that I've already mentioned, getting me away from the physical labor and working around my appointment schedules. That notwithstanding, people were surprised pretty regularly that I kept a job during treatment. I ran into my cousin online in my 9th week, we got to chatting and she was surprised, as a clinical psychologist, that I was still working, and that kinda got me thinking.

Now if you haven't gotten it yet, I'm stubborn. Once I set a course of action it's difficult for me to change that course. I've gotten better in the last few years, but still see that as one of my more consistent behaviors. When I put this in motion, I was determined to work for the duration. Part of it (a damn big part of it) was I couldn't afford it on my own, particularly if I wasn't working. Some of you may not understand this, but deciding between being on a donor list or state assistance would be a rough decision for me, that's how much I am against any state or federal assistance. I realize that may be pretty pointed to some folks, but please remember, this whole mess you're reading is just my opinion, don't let that put you off!

So I feel like at this point I'm in a catch-22. I have to work full time to maintain my benefits, and in the last couple of weeks it's progressively harder. Not "Geez, I don't think I can work today I should stay home", nothing quite that simple to quash.

By the second or third week of treatment, I recognized I started the week pretty good, then slowly kind of lost my giddeup through the week, and by Friday afternoon I was ready for a couple of days recuperation. As I got further into the treatment, by Thursday afternoon I was ready for the weekend but managed to grind through Friday without too much effort.

The last couple of weeks have been different, though. Again, we're back to the inconsistencies of the side effects. Last week, by Thursday I was pretty much done, finished the week alright and still had a decent evening Friday before turning in. This week, by Wednesday I was done, Thursday and Friday have been more zombie than anything else, and as a bonus I've been visited with nausea from hell and diarrhea from hell's version of hell.

One of the things that have really been made evident to me is I'm a faker. During this treatment, just like in my life before it, if I was sick or under the weather you only knew it if you really knew me or I let you know it. That's not bragging, it's just the type

79

of person I am. Now I know (or *think* I know) the side effects are pretty much beyond my control. You know, even as I'm writing that I wonder how correct that is. Anyway, last weekend I had my kids here, and when my kids are here, in treatment or not, I have to be pretty bad off before I can't put a bright face on it, and they never know.

One of the questions Kathleen had for me when I first reported the loss of appetite and nausea was if I was queasy or actually throwing up. Well, this far into it I've avoided the indignity of worshiping at the porcelain altar, but it's been a close thing sometimes. The only thing I can really tell you is whenever all that was active, I always knew where the closest bathroom was and ate a lot of mint. Didn't seem to matter what form it came in, tea or breath mints or gum or Junior Mints, as long as it was mint. That really helped my stomach, the only qualifier was at its worst, I avoided the Junior Mints. The chocolate coating was what I was really avoiding.

So tonight's my 11th shot. Wish me luck, and since you've been this far with me, thank you. If you're at about the same place in your treatment, congratulations! Don't feel like you're the only one who's gotten this far and just thought "Fuck it. It aint worth it, I want my life back, I want my appetite back, I want to sleep a straight eight without drugging myself, I'm had enough and I'm DONE!" I'm there with you, brother (or sister), keep the faith and I'll do the same. If you haven't tried journaling, this might be a time to consider it. All I know is banging my frustrations into my laptop keyboard has helped keep me sane and taking the next shot when it's the last thing I want to think about.

My 12th week results don't really hold any surprises, as you'll see on the next page.

XV

Date: 4·23○8
Tx Week: 13
Rx: Gemzyp 180 ... Friday
RBV 2 pills BID

Since your last visit, have you had any of the following?
- ☐ Chest pain
- ☒ Shortness of breath
- ☒ Dizziness
- ☒ Cough
- ☒ Fatigue
- ☒ Fever

- ☐ Rash
- ☐ Vision changes
- ☒ Mood changes
- ☐ New medical condition
- ☒ Pain issues
- ☒ Sleep problems

- ☐ Heartburn
- ☒ Nausea
- ☐ Vomiting
- ☐ Appetite changes
- ☐ Weight loss/gain

5'8
2/3

Explain:

Since your last visit please rate the following:

Current energy level:	0 1 2 ③ 4 5 6 7 8 9 10	(0 = Bed bound -- 10 = Normal)
Irritability	0 1 2 3 4 5 6 7 ⑧ 9 10	(0 = None at all -- 10 = Extreme)
Anger	0 1 2 3 4 5 6 ⑦ 8 9 10	(0 = None at all -- 10 = Extreme)
Depression	0 ① 2 3 4 5 6 7 8 9 10	(0 =None at all -- 10 = Extreme)
Thoughts of self-injury	⓪ 1 2 3 4 5 6 7 8 9 10	(0 = Never -- 10 = Constantly)
Thoughts of harming others	⓪ 1 2 3 4 5 6 7 8 9 10	(0 = Never -- 10 = Constantly)
Family/Social support	0 1 2 3 4 5 6 7 8 9 ⑩	(0 = No support -- 10 = Excellent support)

Work status: ☒ Working ☐ Not working ☐ Retired ☐ Work restriction _____

Patient concerns or questions:
1. Headaches, Joint Pain, Fatigue/Stamina Level
2.
3.
Using all of acetaminophen everyday usually for head

*******************************For clinic use only below this line*******************************

Wants to know can he use aleve.
also has had off and on week of
generic Vicodan - knoll - has been wone
nearly one per day - general body
aches

Recommendations:
1. _____
2. _____
3. _____

bs tnc:0903

82

Let me interpret some of this for you. Under my laundry list of side effects I've been experiencing, I noted I've lost around 15 pounds (most due to cutting 1,500-2,500 calories/day out of the beer diet!). This was due to a lighter appetite along with alcohol intake.

Fatigue, dizziness and shortness of breath started showing up by my 6th or 8th week, but by now it was a concern as my job up to this point was primarily manual labor. If you compare the number scales to my original sheet, it's obvious the treatment is having an effect just about body-wide, from energy to sleep to thought processes. Also, just as I was warned, irritability and anger were up a bit.

All that being said, these effects were going to be experienced by me either way. One thing I've always believed is attitude makes an incredible difference every single day, and this is no different. Feeling like crap or on top of the world, I've always been able to put a genuine smile on. For my Gastro Girls, even though I was accurate and forthcoming with my symptoms, I could always do it with humor and a smile, even if it was temporary.

Nothing else really stands out in that first couple of months that I haven't already mentioned except for depression. My nurses had me fill out a "Depression Scale" in April, June and August to track how I was reacting emotionally to treatment.

This first scale gives you a baseline, but a true baseline would be from before treatment started. I did one of those with a pre-treatment mindset and my total score was 2. Compare that with the next chart and you'll get an idea of the impact the medication was starting to have.

DEPRESSION SCALE

Circle the number for each statement which best describes how often you felt or behaved this way during the past week:

Chandler
4-23

	During the past week:	Rarely or None of the Time (Less than 1 day)	Some or a Little of the Time (1-2 days)	Occasionally or a Moderate Amount of Time (3-4 days)	Most or All of the Time (5-7 days)
1	I was bothered by things that usually don't bother me.	0	1	2	3
2	I did not feel like eating; my appetite was poor.	0	1	2	3
3	I felt that I could not shake off the blues even with the help from my family or friends.	0	1	2	3
4	I felt that I was just as good as other people.	3	2	1	0
5	I had trouble keeping my mind on what I was doing.	0	1	2	3
6	I felt depressed.	0	1	2	3
7	I felt that everything I did was an effort.	0	1	2	3
8	I felt hopeful about the future.	3	2	1	0
9	I thought my life had been a failure.	0	1	2	3
10	I felt fearful.	0	1	2	3
11	My sleep was restless.	0	1	2	3
12	I was happy.	3	2	1	0
13	I talked less than usual.	0	1	2	3
14	I felt lonely.	0	1	2	3
15	People were unfriendly.	0	1	2	3
16	I enjoyed life.	3	2	1	0
17	I had crying spells.	0	1	2	3
18	I felt sad.	0	1	2	3
19	I felt that people disliked me.	0	1	2	3
20	I could not get "going."	0	1	2	3

TOTAL SCORE: 0   3   8   3

(14)

During most of this treatment I've maintained well enough that most folks aren't aware I'm in treatment, which I'm grateful for. I have never been one to really need anyone's sympathy or comfort when sick.

My roommate and I go back quite awhile, and have lots of water, booze and tears under the bridge at one time or another. We're both what we call "aware", we sense others mood, feelings, hidden agendas and secrets with remarkable accuracy. With each other, for the most part, we're open books, since we're both aware and have been through so much together.

That being said, when I don't feel good I insulate. I don't want anyone to touch me, sympathize with me, or even look at me very hard. I put myself into a shell, a cave, choose your metaphor, I withdraw and handle my malady and everything's better. Right or wrong, that's how I deal with pain, sickness and discomfort.

My roommate realizes this, and being as close as we are, sometimes can't take it. Seeing someone you love in pain is miserable, seeing and feeling it in your soul is worse, and we find it's easier sometimes to kick down the others wall, barge in and comfort them, their feelings be damned. Honestly it's partly selfish relief of the pressure, but it's also because the one of us doing okay knows it's the best thing for the recipient, whether they know it or not.

With all that background, here's what I started seeing in about the eighth week, although it had been going on throughout treatment. It had gradually gotten intense enough that I finally recognized it, that's all. Midweek after my 11th shot I had a day. No rhyme or reason, just got up feeling questionable and slowly deteriorated through the day. The difference was, this time I was talking with a lady that I can *talk* with, that's on my and my roommates spiritual, metaphysical-type level, and I started realizing that some of our conversation put me on the verge of tears. I'm well aware of my emotions, but crying isn't something that's one of my defaults, okay? But damn, we were listening to some Jimmy Buffett and talking and there were times I had to bury myself in my computer screen, what the hell? Being who I am, I had to closet it, then take it all out later to dissect all that emotion. It shouldn't have surprised me, some of the potential side effects are depression and irritability, so high emotion shouldn't surprise me, but it did. Just another bonus of treatment, even if you're an emotional rock, don't be surprised if your rock is a little like soapstone for six months.

XVI

Well, time for some good news! I'm almost halfway through, and had my follow-up ophthalmologist appointment today. Let me give you some history and some recent side effects to set the stage, alright?

For some reason I've always been protective of my eyes. I say that like it's the exception to the rule, and sometimes it seems to be. Obviously I didn't mind abusing my liver on a wholesale scale for years with alcohol, drugs or a combination of both. By the same token, I've pretty consistently taken vitamin, mineral and herb supplements since my early twenties, so it's kind of a dichotomy. It's almost like on one level I was aware of the risk I was putting myself at, and trying to fix it on the back side, nullifying (or nearly so) both efforts. I'm sure a psychologist somewhere would have a hay day with me if he could just get me to lie still long enough.

But my eyes seem to be the exception. I've always been cautious with my eye health, and have worked plenty of jobs where risks were high. Protective gear, welding or cutting goggles, and just being aware of reactions have always been second nature to me concerning my eyes. I've spent a lifetime avoiding injury to my eyes, then voluntarily injured them to correct my vision, but that one instance was carefully investigated and studied before I decided to have the Lasik done. Who knows, maybe my eyes were burned from my head in a former life and it's a carryover (wow, where'd that come from?).

Like I mentioned earlier, an eye exam was required before I could start the interferon treatment, so I logically assumed there would be some risk to my eyes. Again, with proper observation I felt it was an acceptable risk. As I mentioned earlier, seven or eight weeks into the treatment, I started noticing a new side effect. My shots were Friday, I slept through the worst of the side effects, but in the seventh week my eyes were sore on Saturday, bad enough to want nothing other than sunglasses and closed eyelids for an hour or more.

It seems the theme to this whole rant has been partially focused on the inconsistency of side effects, doesn't it? I handled it the seventh weekend, and by the time I woke up on Sunday my eyes seemed fine. I stayed aware of my eyes the following week, and noticed I was more light sensitive, and by the end of the day sometimes the ache would return, although not at the same level as the weekend. Of course, it wasn't that way every day, that would be way too easy to predict.

One thing that was consistent was the next few weekends, I had the same reaction on Saturday and then into Sunday. The closest I've gotten to describing it is a headache in my eyes. You know how a headache can range from irritating to incapacitating for no particular reason? That's kind of how my eyes were, somewhere in that range, sometimes so minor I'd almost forget about it and sometimes bad enough I couldn't even read or watch an episode of Firefly. If I can't watch an episode of Firefly it's pretty major juju, just for your personal scale.

Since it was manageable, I didn't call out the troops. I had an eye appointment coming up, so we dealt with it for three shot cycles. It continued to escalate, however, which concerned me a bit. Not necessarily worse, but longer duration, lasting well into Sunday by my 11th shot.

That's where the good news comes in! My appointment went fine today, nothing to be concerned with, so that's a relief. I had a good Q&A with my ophthalmologist, and it put my eye health concerns to rest and made me start thinking in another direction.

I think I've mentioned the Zicam, the stuffy nose and headaches. Well, maybe those side effects and my eyes are all tied together! If you think about it, physically they are, with the nasal and sinus passages. That was something I hadn't even considered.

I'll watch closer the next shot, 'cause I don't recall if my sinuses are worse right after the shot, but I know I'm more prone to headaches then, so maybe the eye discomfort is hand in hand with sinus hatefulness, eh? I don't understand why pain or discomfort is easier for me to deal with when I know the source of it, but that's the way it is.

Actually...hmmmm...I do understand that. Once I know the source, I know if it's something temporary or something I need to address with bigger guns, whether it's treatable or not, and having that knowledge would give anyone some comfort. I have an appointment with Dr S next week, so he's got some 'splainin to do, Lucy. If the interferon tends to irritate or swell the sinuses, especially if it's cumulative, that would explain a lot, and give me a benchmark for expectations during the second half of treatment. If this is going to escalate, well that could get very interesting over the next 12 weeks. Of course, I'm using "interesting" in a purely sado-masochistic, "what the hell is he talking about?", please-sir-can-I-have-another-beating manner.

So we've gotten by that part safely. I'll take this opportunity to give you a warning, kiddies. When I had my first shot, Kathleen covered a lot of ground with me concerning side effects, possible other meds I could end up on, all that stuff. At the same time we scheduled blood work for the entire treatment period, and she went over some high points on that.

One of her warnings (more like motherly advice) was if I missed a blood work date, they'd give me a couple of days and then be calling me. I'm not a big schedule freak, don't put reminders on every electronic gadget I own, but this was important to me, so I made every lab visit on time. Every one, that is, except my 12th week.

At first it was weekly, then semi-weekly, then monthly. I made every one up to my eighth week I think, but then had a month break. My schedule was on Tuesdays for lab samples, and Wednesday of my 12th week I had a call from Pam midmorning. It had gone to voicemail, and I returned the call as soon as I heard the message, a little frustrated that I'd made it this far and then missed one.

Your blood will be drawn before you start treatment to establish a baseline. The focus (to my layman eyes) seems to be red and white blood cell counts, pregnancy, and viral level or load. Since I was blessed with external plumbing, I don't think they concentrated too much on the pregnancy part, but the rest was rigidly monitored. Just FYI, if you haven't gotten to week 12 yet, this was the sample taken before my midway appointment, and the biggie on this sample was viral load, which tells my staff how well I'm responding to the treatment.

Here's another of the backward tattoos for reading in the mirror…**Don't miss this bloodwork!** I had Pam corner me and come the closest yet to demanding something of me, damnit, more blood right flipping now! Nah, my Girls wouldn't do that to me, but I was frustrated enough I went to the clinic after work that day and got the blood drawn. Pam did remind me of the tests they would run on this for input at my next appointment, and really I think any other time I'd have gotten away with Thursday or Friday before I got a call, but this one was the biggest test so far, with an appointment following soon after.

I know you're probably tired of hearing it by now, but you need a great relationship with your Gastro Girls, they'll keep you on the path sometimes when no one else can.

XVII

So, the 12th shot is out of the way, I'm entering my 13th week, and my biggie appointment with 'the team' is done. Interesting stuff, that appointment was.

First off, when Pam called to remind me I owed them body fluids for their nefarious tests, we talked about any appointments scheduled. She mentioned the next appointment was on "bring your nurse a cookie" day, known by some as Administrative Professionals Day. We got a laugh out of that, she set me straight on any other commitments I had and that was that.

When that Wednesday rolled around, I went by our local market and got two of the biggest cookies I could find. These weren't the Mrs. Fields pizza-size cookies, but they were the size of a small salad plate, anyway. All I knew is they were a helluva lot bigger than I'd want to eat.

I snuck those into my exam room (I thought), but when Kathleen came in she zoned right in on the treats, laughing about it. After the general symptom and side effects discussion, she left and Pam was in there two minutes later. I honestly don't think they talked when Kathleen left, but I have a great relationship with my Gastro Girls, and when they know I'll be in, the one not handling my appointment always stops by to do her own interview. I appreciate this, and love the relationship that drives that behavior.

Anyway, I thought Pam was going to cry when she saw her cookie. We hugged, did the whole mini-interview regarding treatment, and Dr S arrived to throw his two cents in.

Here's something that may seem off, but I have to make you aware of it. My regular doctor, Dr K, is a great general practitioner. I don't know what his specialty is if any, but he's suited great for what he does. Dr S, on the other hand, is a specialist whose only focus is getting your liver and blood disorder fixed.

That being said, in our discussion during this appointment, we went over medications I was taking for the HepC and for the side effects. As I was detailing what some dosages were to handle side effects he started losing his mind a bit. Now I've already outlined with you my occasional doses of pain killers etc to handle side effects, but when I told Dr S he was a bit spun up.

My nurses originally limited me to 2000mg of acetaminophen, which is in Tylenol. What I didn't realize was the same pain killer is in Vicodin, so on the days when Tylenol wasn't doing the job I would take 1-2 Vicodin also. On a normal day I was taking a couple Tylenol sometime late morning if necessary (usually), and two Tylenol PM with my evening dose, so my 2000mg was taken most days.

Okay, back to Dr S. Please don't misunderstand this, I'm in no way disappointed or dissatisfied with either of my doctors, they're doing the separate jobs they have trained for, and they're doing one helluva job in my opinion. When Dr S heard my side effects treatment during this appointment, he told me flat out "My goal is not for you to be pain-free during this treatment, my goal is to kill the HepC you have, and if that means you have to have headaches sometimes you're going to have to knuckle under and take it." Not the best bedside manner, but really should he have that? Not in these circumstances, I think. He's treating people for an active, aggressive disease that could eventually kill them, and in his opinion if the treatments side effects are unpleasant, well buck up buttercup!

I understand where he's coming from and appreciate it. But like my mom and my Gastro Girls,

I didn't listen and follow blindly in this case either. Yes, did you hear the disclaimer coming?

I listened to my doctor, and after that appointment let side effects go further without medicating. But I also listened to my body. Yes, sometimes I treated the discomfort early and maybe unnecessarily, and I understand that. However, I also knew from experience that my tolerance for pain killers is high, and that sometimes if these side effects weren't treated they would temporarily take me out. When that happened, the reaction of my body couldn't help support the HepC treatment, in my opinion. So the short version is I listened to my doctor, and followed what he said balanced against my own body's needs.

I've harped on both the relationship with your staff and your relationship with your body, and have been blessed with two great communication systems. I've continued to treat my symptoms as I see fit while taking his opinion into account. Once again, I'm not recommending this as your path of treatment, it's what worked for me, that's all.

With that being said, I've been experiencing sinus problems for the entire 12 weeks, pretty consistently. Recently, my jaw has begun aching at the joint on my left side only. It's enough pain that it's good it's just one side! We talked about this during my appointment, or more accurately the "reunion". That's kind of what it was, with me and my support lady, then Kathleen, then she left and Pam came in, then Kathleen returned and finally Dr S showed up. While all of us were chatting it up crammed into this little examination room, my jaw ache was discussed.

Dr S never really said anything about it, concentrating instead on my treatment numbers (which were good) and my treatment of side effects. While Kathleen, he and I were talking about that, I noticed Pam stepped away and was in an intense, whispered conversation with my support lady. What I found out later was Pam told her I needed to go to my regular doctor and get something for what had all the earmarks of a sinus infection. Pam mentioned that Dr S and the GI clinic didn't really treat anything beyond the HepC, so treatment of other symptoms would be up to my primary care physician or specialists such as ophthalmologists, dermatologists, etc depending on the symptom.

We needed to hear that bluntly to make us aware the GI clinic wasn't as concerned with my overall health as they were my response to the treatment. This can be frustrating, given that you've signed on for the treatment through the GI clinic, but have to go to other doctors to treat the side effects of the Pegasys and Ribavirin. Especially when you're already tired and irritable and nauseated and...you get the picture.

In talking with my nurses after the treatment, this is something that bears repeating. The GI clinic and doctor are focused on the treatment and your liver. In addition, your nurses are monitoring your overall health, but they may be forced to refer you to another physician or clinic that can address the maladies brought on by the treatment.

That may sound harsh, but that's their job, and by having a good relationship with my Gals, Pam was comfortable enough to take my support lady aside and make us aware of their focus and what I should do regarding the "other effects". I truly hope you have as good or a better relationship with your staff. Your treatment will be so much more comfortable knowing someone's in charge that actually cares about you, your treatment and your overall health.

XVIII

Another side effect I had to finally submit to was dry skin. Remember, I'm a guy, and primarily lotion use isn't for skin health in most guys opinion. At least that's been my experience, but when I went to my first appointment Kathleen warned me I may notice more dry skin and have to use lotion more consistently. I took that in, mentally agreeing to use at least as much lotion in the future six months as I had in the past six months. That wasn't real hard, since I hadn't used any in probably the last year.

My support lady has been in the cosmetology industry off and on for the last twenty years. She's been a stylist, trainer, instructor, owner, manager, blah blah blah. Suffice to say she's very aware of fashions, personal hygiene and health, grooming, all that happy stuff. Three months into treatment, she started noticing me lightly scratching, and during my appointment the staff noticed my skin was dryer and I had a light rash in several areas.

Of course, this led to my support cornering me with a lotion bottle soon after, and I did notice a difference. So if you're like me and never use lotion, plan on a change during treatment. I can't guarantee you'll have the same result, but I would suggest having some lotion available, and if you notice yourself unusually itchy and being able to find an orgasmic sweet spot that you never got from scratching before, maybe some lotion would be in order?

Here's the physiology attached to it, which I found out later. Your liver processes bile. Your bile level colors your feces and urine when it's being processed correctly. Another substance is bile salt, which your liver also processes *when it's able to*. When it's not able to process bile, your feces gets pale, your urine gets colorless, and the bile salt tends to come out your pores with sweat and oil. When that salt is on your skin it tends to make you dry out and itch. There will be some more discussion on this in post-treatment for you and I both.

These were all things that came up during or around my 12th week checkup. Overall it was a good checkup, with reasonable results and side effects. The only thing that mildly concerns me is if these side effects are going to act cumulatively, getting more intense during the last three months as poison levels in my body go up.

I've discussed this with my staff, who didn't have a firm answer for me either way. This doesn't surprise me, since the side effects are so inconsistent from one patient to another. I was told at the first appointment side effects would range somewhere between almost nothing to incapacitation for six months depending on the person, and even the same person could have radically different side effects day to day. Well, all that was accurate, so we'll just monitor it and I'll refer back in this journal and I guess you and I will see, eh?

XIX

I suppose it's time for soul bearing again. It has been 10 days since my last appointment, I took my 14th shot two days ago, and it seems it's been a time of realizations and epiphanies.

First off, let's talk about meds, and my cavalier use of different medications. In retrospect I'm glad I put so many disclosures into the text before this. You'll see why as we go on.

Let me refresh your memory with this. It'll help me keep things in perspective also. After talking with Dr S, I kind of ignored his reaction to my painkiller medicating initially. However, I continued to think about it a little here and a little there, until a firm realization started to gel. It's funny how different, seemingly unrelated occurrences can shape and influence your decisions.

As I mentioned earlier, I backed off the Tylenol after my appointment. I "knuckled down" as Dr S said, and cut the aspirin by more than half. I also wasn't quite as freehanded with the Vicodins and managed to survive. Here was the real mind blower, though.

I've mentioned the Zicam that I was on a multi-daily use for my sinuses, which I thought had also led to a sinus infection. I had tickets for a concert on Sunday night five days after my appointment, and on that afternoon ended up 2/3rds of the way to Seattle before I realized I hadn't brought any Zicam. The concert started at 7PM, and since I was going downtown early I had brought Ribavirin and PM Tylenol, but no Zicam or Benadryl. Once I noticed this I decided it was something I could survive and went about my planned day and evening in the city.

This is one of those cases of preparing for your day and going about it, symptoms be damned. It worked out well, I noticed a bit of congestion but nothing that didn't pass fairly quickly. By the end of the evening, I decided my Zicam use may have been a bit overboard, and knew Dr S wouldn't mind me backing off even something as innocent as a nasal inhaler.

Since then it's been a week and I haven't used Zicam at all. At the same time I decided it was time for some other experimentation, but this time the kind my staff would more likely approve of.

Every evening up to this point I was taking 2 Ribavirin, 2 Tylenol PM, and 2 Benadryl. Still plagued by headaches, I changed my dosage to just the Ribavirin and Tylenol, thinking the Tylenol-free benefit may be offset by a lack of sleep and the 2 tablets would be within my limits for the day anyway. To my surprise, the lack of Benadryl and Zicam didn't have any negative effect on my sinuses or my sleep. Actually it seemed just the opposite.

So there was my first revelation, that my almost kneejerk reaction to sinus congestion wasn't necessarily wrong, but after 12 weeks it was time to have some restraint. As much as I hate to admit it, Dr S was right! The crazy thing was not only was I not using Zicam, but after rolling it over in my mind, I started thinking maybe that was part of the problem. I'd been dosing with Zicam two to five times per day for over eleven weeks, and maybe my sinuses were just pissed off by this time. It sure seemed that may be the case, after several clear schnozz days.

I hadn't done anything thus far about the possible sinus infection. Those symptoms hadn't improved, but I was hesitant to add another chemical into the soup I already had simmering. Remember the colloidal silver I had used for treatment? Silver is a potent anti-bacterial, so before I checked the infection out I decided on an experiment. I started drinking between eight and 24 ounces of water daily with colloidal silver, a concoction we call "witch water". I also started drinking the juice of a full fresh lemon at least daily mixed with filtered water, the citric acid being another great antibacterial. Please hear this loud and clear...here it comes, the disclaimer...*I don't know for sure these two naturopathic treatments did a damn thing!* All I know is that in a week my jaw wasn't stiff, and my sinuses had stayed clearer than they'd been in 2 months, and I didn't have to get prescription antibiotics to make it work.

Another bonus it took me a few days to recognize was that my eyes weren't aching as much. I was still pretty light sensitive all the time, but the "headache in my eyes" seemed to dissipate. Do you think stopping the Zicam and letting my sinuses get back to a normal size may have helped?

Between those two my jaw stopped hurting in less than a week. Remember, I'm my own best doctor as far as I'm concerned, so again, I don't recommend you do any of this without careful consideration. This seemed to work for me, but unless you've been treating your body as long as I have I'd recommend you check out any of these options carefully before just setting sail on the good ship DrSteve with me.

The last huge thing that came to my attention is much more spiritual. Until about 12 years ago I was what you might consider a holy roller or a devout religious man, depending on your perspective regarding organized religion.

Whichever way you see it, you get the idea where I was at spiritually. But 10 to 12 years ago I became disillusioned with organized religion. I completely walked away from organized religion, and extensively checked out options to the standard Judeo-Christian system. One of the things I became aware of was my own spiritual energy, and over several years learned to monitor where my energy was being spent wisely or wasted. The reason I bring this up is tied in with my Sunday concert night.

Being in touch with my body, I had realized over the weeks that getting upset about something would temporarily take me out pretty quickly. Let me give you a little more history so you know where

I'm coming from, and maybe recognize a little of yourself in here too.

By the time I was 14, I still hadn't topped 4'10". My mom, when I was preteen, sometimes referred to me as her bantam rooster, because my older bigger brothers would pester me to a certain point, where I would eventually lose it and attack, regardless the cost or size difference.

By the time I hit my teens, I had started getting my temper under control. In my freshman year I sprouted ten inches. I refer to that as the Year of the Highwaters. You won't find the year mentioned in any Japanese calendars, like the Year of the Rat, but it's just as pivotal to me sometimes.

So I've never gotten real big, and had my temper in some semblance of control. I still went nuclear occasionally, but not very often. As the years went by the occurrences were less, and by the time I started treatment it was reasonably rare. However, once treatment started I recognized the necessity of guarding my energy jealously.

All of this leads to Sunday at the concert.

I realize this might not be your cup of tea, but I got turned on several years ago to a guy named Mike Doughty, who used to be with Soul Coughing. He had a concert with The BoDeans in Seattle about halfway through my treatment and I decided I had no choice but to go.

This was the concert I forgot my Zicam for. Here's the cool thing, I got to Seattle, hung out awhile downtown, and by the time I headed into the concert hall I was feeling a bit of the fatigue I'd been plagued with for the last few months. I decided to just go with it, if there was a price to be paid I'd have to decide the next day if it'd been worth it or not.

I don't go to very many concerts, even before treatment. This one I was very excited about, the venue a small theater that had been built in 1907, so it was comparatively a cozy venue. Also, being built that long ago, there were plenty of narrow steep stairways to navigate. Once in my seat I was content to hang out and wait for the show to begin.

As I said, maybe this isn't your cup of tea, but the show was incredible. This is my own interpretation and my own emotions, but the energy level Mike's band put out was phenomenal. I was jazzed by all the songs, familiar to me, and felt like I was on the best adrenaline high I'd ever experienced. I don't pretend to understand this, but their energy level I simply fed from. I don't know how I identified the source, but at the time I knew it was from the band, not the crowd.

Later the way I verified it was when the second band came out. The BoDeans were great, I enjoyed their show, but honestly I'd have taken two Mike Doughty shows instead, the energy was that amazing during the first show.

During the second show we had a lady in front of us that was very much into the BoDeans. I can't blame her for that, but she was continuously standing up or sitting on the edge of her folded chair, blocking the view for a few rows behind her. At first I got irritated, and it kept building as the show went on and she kept blocking my view. I thought it through and realized I was allowing this lady to drain the energy I had 'stored' during Mike's opening act. Once I was aware of that, I stopped the energy drain

After the show, I felt like a new man. Here it was, after ten PM, about an hour after my normal treatment bedtime, and driving home was a breeze.

But the universe really wanted to test my newfound control one more time.

About a mile from home I stopped at a grocery store. I set down my keys, dug pills out, took them and then went into the store. I'd waited to take pills until I was close to home so if the sleeping pills kicked in quick I wasn't fighting to stay awake while driving.

Leaving the store I checked the pocket my keys are always in, and had done a full pat-down of all pockets by the time I'd gotten to the car. Then I realized I hadn't picked up my keys after taking meds.

So here we are, after 11 PM by now, strolling over to one of the light poles in the parking lot to call the tow company's number posted there. It was about an hour wait, during which time I could have gotten myself into a full-on fit (and would have, in the pre-treatment Steve mode). But the evening had stuck with me, what I'd experienced at the concert, and I managed to enjoy myself. All the bright sides were there – I had a jacket, the temperature was alright, it wasn't raining, my symptoms were pretty stable, all in all it could have been *much* worse.

One of the things I realized during this time was kind of a backhand present from the gods. In going through treatment, I was learning through necessity to control my moods better. Guess it just underlines that everything happens for a reason, and you can find some good in any situation.

XX

What a vacation! Actually, I've taken a few weeks away from this as a necessity. Although I love writing, and this has helped me to "vent", I had to break for a bit due to the treatment, partially.

I'm in my 18th week, so it's been almost six weeks since I've been here. During that time symptoms have continued, but things may be cumulative.

Things haven't gotten worse necessarily, but have seemed to accumulate. The general fatigue, nausea etc have continued, but once past the halfway mark have seemed to intensify. The irritation has also acquired a shorter fuse.

Early on some of my irritation stemmed from sensitivity to touch.

Part II

<u>XXI</u>

That may seem like a strange place to leave off on the last page, but there's a reason for it.

I was writing during my 14th week about the concert, then suddenly was writing in the 18th week, and you can see how that sort of broke off abruptly. That all ties into a neat little package.

The first part of this book was written as it happened for the most part. I would sit down a few times each week and throw my impressions of the week at my laptop, and it stayed in pretty good order. However, by the time I got to the 14th week, maintaining daily activity was turning into a challenge. I had a bright spot in my 18th week, and then everything kind of closed down. I kept a historical record up until then, and realistically, after that I just didn't give a damn.

115

Let me give you an idea of where I was at mentally, emotionally and physically.

I tried to keep a diary of sorts with noteworthy events after the 14th week. When I look back at that now, there are two entries. One is from mid-June and is basically worthless. The other is from the first of August *almost a month after treatment was finished.* The entry starts with "August 1…Rage, just fucking rage…" , well, so much for noteworthy events.

Actually it does help some though. That rage only made it to the computer, not into my life or to the ones I care about. Obviously the lessons I'd learned months earlier were paying off, and I could still reign in the crazy emotions the residual medication was causing.

So mentally I wasn't too bad off, emotionally I was on a tightrope at times, and physically, well, that was a whole other issue.

Just to help you understand and me to keep this in perspective, the chronological record I was keeping ended the 14th week. Basically, the balance

116

of this book has been written post-treatment starting
about a month after treatment was completed. That's
not a spoiler, kiddies, if you have any awareness of
personalities you already know I completed the damn
treatment....

XXII

My 18th week was the first week in June. By that time it was difficult to hold thoughts for very long, I couldn't follow a movie beginning to end, reading was a sad, sad joke, and my memory I couldn't remember having.

Here's what my outlook on paper was from an appointment the second week in June:

DEPRESSION SCALE

Circle the number for each statement which best describes how often you felt or behaved this way during the past week:

Chandler 6-11-'08

	During the past week:	Rarely or None of the Time (Less than 1 day)	Some or a Little of the Time (1-2 days)	Occasionally or a Moderate Amount of Time (3-4 days)	Most or All of the Time (5-7 days)
1	I was bothered by things that usually don't bother me.	0	1	(2)	3
2	I did not feel like eating; my appetite was poor.	0	1	2	(3)
3	I felt that I could not shake off the blues even with the help from my family or friends.	(0)	1	2	3
4	I felt that I was just as good as other people.	3	2	1	(0)
5	I had trouble keeping my mind on what I was doing.	0	1	(2)	3
6	I felt depressed.	0	(1)	2	3
7	I felt that everything I did was an effort.	0	1	(2)	3
8	I felt hopeful about the future.	3	2	1	(0)
9	I thought my life had been a failure.	0	(1)	2	3
10	I felt fearful.	(0)	1	2	3
11	My sleep was restless.	0	1	(2)	3
12	I was happy.	3	2	1	(0)
13	I talked less than usual.	0	1	(2)	3
14	I felt lonely.	(0)	1	2	3
15	People were unfriendly.	0	(1)	2	3
16	I enjoyed life.	3	2	1	(0)
17	I had crying spells.	(0)	1	2	3
18	I felt sad.	0	(1)	2	3
19	I felt that people disliked me.	(0)	1	2	3
20	I could not get "going."	0	1	(2)	3

TOTAL SCORE: (19)   4   12   3

My last scale like this was a 14, the one before that a 2 before treatment. Yeah, looking back on this paperwork I can see where I was in a downward spiral.

My appointment was kind of reflective of these forms. Sitting on the exam table, the first thing Pam asked me about was my posture. I realized then I was hunched forward and down, and breathing shallow with a light persistent cough.

We talked for a bit, her getting an idea of how things had been since my last visit. She got most of the truth from me, but if I started sugar-coating anything my support lady was right there to give her the straight scoop. Like a good clinician, Pam was hearing what she was seeing of me more than she was hearing what I was saying.

Dr. S came in and did his thing and obviously didn't like what he was seeing and hearing either. He came back to the fact over and over that I only had 5 weeks left, just hang in there, all that happy crap.

While Dr S and I were talking, Pam and my support lady were again in a whispered conversation. Even as physically shattered as I was, I could see whatever their conversation entailed, it wasn't good for me.

After Dr. S left, Pam was suddenly in my grill. Not in a bad way, but right up on me with "You can't quit, you've only got five weeks, you've been such a trooper so far just buck up for another little while." She was fairly emotional at the time, and I didn't realize all of why until later.

It was actually two things that got her. The first was her conversation with my support lady. They were ordering a chest x-ray that morning, and if it came back even questionable they were hospitalizing me. She (and Dr S) were concerned over my breathing, consistent cough, and posture, and thought there may be a problem in my lungs that my body couldn't fight, being in its weakened state from the hep-c medication. Remember, the treatment gives your immune system a whammy, and since I'd lost my spleen in 1999, that was a double-whammy on the immune system.

The second reason was more emotional. We'd been fighting this for over 18 weeks and my symptoms, in the big picture, had been manageable if not minimal. However, they were seeing me now under the influence of worsening symptoms, and I think they see a lot of people quit when the symptoms really start taking toll. During treatment, they've formed a "cheerleader" bond that has to make it difficult to see their subjects do either one, hurt or quit. I can understand quitting intellectually, but not personally. My roommate kept telling her "He's gone this far, he's not going to quit, Pam." I told her this far in, I'd finish the regimen if I had to do it on my hands and knees.

That wasn't the only why, though. Those folks see their patients literally go through hell, and I'm sure it's disheartening to them to see a patient go part of the distance and then not be able to maintain. Please hear me accurate, I'm not beating my chest, and I'm not judging the folks that can't finish the treatment the first time (or second, or third). I'm well aware that folks have had it better and worse than I have, I'm just thankful that I could finish the regimen. But these nurses carry your load with you the whole way, and I'm sure it breaks their hearts to see someone go part of the distance and hurt so bad they have to quit.

I've always been articulate, love a good war with words, and describe things in a way that just sucks people along with wherever I'm going. During this time, however, just communicating verbally was one of my biggest challenges. Not necessarily communicating, but communicating the way I was used to. I'd be talking along, in the midst of explaining something fairly complex or involved, and just lose the next word I knew belonged there. If I lost the word long enough, or couldn't remember a synonym that would fit almost as well, I'd lose where the conversation was going completely.

Holy crap! The description I started using was my mind was like swiss cheese. I warned my kids to be careful with plans. If they made plans and I agreed to them, remind me of the plans a day or two before. I made this warning after calling my daughter to find out why she wasn't ready to be picked up for a weekend visit and she reminded me she had to raincheck that weekend. Yes, she'd told me that at the beginning of the week, and by Friday it wasn't even a vague memory.

At work I had to keep a notepad nearby at all times. If something came up that interrupted my ailing train of thought I'd have to note what I was doing or it may never get returned to.

Physically I thought I was doing alright, all things considered. I would make it through the week and recuperate on the weekends, just like early in treatment. What I didn't realize was how others were seeing me. My support lady, her family and my family, had a different perspective of me that I didn't know about until after treatment was over in mid-July.

XXIIa

Let me add something in here, in defense of the clinic, Dr S., and the whole staff.

I've said I was fortunate to keep a job during treatment and all that stuff, but a large part of that was due to pure stubbornness, nothing else. That being said, some of my symptoms and reactions were self-inflicted.

My nurses especially were on that from the beginning;

"Steve, have you thought about taking time off?"

"Steve, maybe it's time to cut back on your hours."

"Maybe you'd be better off cutting back your activities."

"You should take it easier during your off times, don't try to do so much."

The reason I added this in here is that while I didn't always listen to my nurses, it wasn't always the best thing to charge straight ahead. Again, this is something you have to decide for yourself and deal with whatever consequences result.

I guess what I'm trying to get across is that the GI doctor and staff and other doctors you see for other symptoms are going to do what they know to do to help you through this, but there are some things you're going to decide to do that will be against their recommendations and wishes. Those decisions will all have results, some miniscule, some minor, and some almost catastrophic.

You're going to have to choose your battles carefully during this treatment. Some, like keeping a job so you have benefits so you can afford to complete the treatment, may be worthwhile. I thought so. But some others, like continuing your physical regimen or trying 'just one drink' probably aren't. Again, it's personal choice, and the only person who can decide if it's worth it is you.

XXIII

Around the middle of June we moved a 3,000 square foot house into storage and a 1,000 square foot house. We were one of the victims of the subprime mortgage debacle, so we stuck things out as long as we could and then moved before the new owners evicted us. I wish there was a kinder way of putting it, but I can't find one even now.

Because of time constraints, it was basically a one-weekend move. Pam heard about this a couple of weeks earlier and immediately talked with my support lady about physical activity. Remember, I'm a stubborn man, and was very active before this whole drama. When there is work to be done, I'm the one you have to take aside and say "Take a break, Trigger, it'll get done"…

Well, not so much in this case. It's funny how things work out, and they always seem to be for the best, depending on your outlook.

———————————

I have three nieces, one which I barely knew until after treatment. The other two are my older brothers daughters, and I'm pretty sure one brings the sun up, the other sets it down in my world. One is the niece I married during treatment (no, I didn't marry her, silly, I officiated her marriage to my favorite nephew-in-law, remember?), the other is a couple of years younger and makes my heart believe in the good in the world.

Megs, the younger one, had a Philippino fiancé, who we met at the wedding of the older niece. Megs asked me a month or so later if they could stay at our place when he deployed to Korea, which he would do from Fairchild AFB. Of course we said yes, but qualified it with 'if we were still in the house'.

Now timing being what it was, he deployed in the beginning of June. Megs saw him off and returned to our house to help us move. It's good the way it worked out, and she was the trooper for us all. Actually, it helped her, being busy after he was gone, and it helped us 'cause she's the type that looks around and says "Uncle Steve, what's next?".

The other thing was my support lady's daughter. We are the same astrological sign, and literally the same personality. The only difference she has that misses being 'real cool' is she's not left-handed. She and her girlfriend weren't living with us, but showed up to lift boxes and shuffle furniture around. I mention this first because they were great help, but second to make a point later. She's *into* me, I can't hide a mood or weakness from her to save my soul, and it will make a huge point later.

We also had most of my kids on and off again to help us move, and overall, it got done. That's really the bottom line, and they were all troopers.

OK, now you've got the basics. We had two trucks, a 12-15 footer from the storage facility, and a 26-footer we got from U-Haul. It seems we made trip after trip after trip, but it wasn't really that way. By Sunday, we had one load in each truck that we were taking to the house, and whatever was left we were taking to storage, dropping off trucks and we were done.

Early on Sunday at the old house, we were taking a breather and my support lady and I were talking. While talking, (yes I was exhausted by then but no one was aware of it) my eyes rolled back into my head for a second, kind of like I was ready to collapse. Well, that was accurate, and while I wasn't going to admit it, she noticed it, of course she did. The remainder of the day I was assigned to pointing, talking, and delegating, and nothing else was allowed by me.

Once we got the house part unloaded (and she kept insisting on taking breaks, what the hell?), we drove to the storage facility to offload the balance and be done. In the house we had a quasi-office with two comfortable chairs. When we reached the storage facility, the chairs were the first thing to come off the truck. I was *forced* into a chair, turned so I could observe the storage area, and relegated to pointing where things should go. What the fuck was she thinking? Actually, if I had to admit it, what she was thinking was "He'll stay in that chair willingly, or there's some duct tape in this storage with his name on it…"

Alright, I'll admit it. With my personality, my support person probably kept me alive through treatment. The move was the ultimate test, in my mind, and because we all survived it, all's good in the world.

Okay, this needs to be repeated. If you're reading this during treatment, you may already have the 'swiss cheese' mind so you've probably forgotten it anyway. My nurses encouraged me over and over to take it easy, slow down, take advantage of medication and treatment that would help me through treatment. I slowed down some, I took some of their medicines, I did some things my way, all in all I survived.

Pam went through this book several times for me. We wanted to keep the flavor of my experience without being too far off medically. Her last comment to me was:

"It's maddening to see people suffer during treatment when there is help. Just like you."

XIV

Let me veer off for a moment, mostly for me. Remember early on I mentioned two car accidents? There's some recall issues that will help us in this.

I mentioned after week 18 my mind was akin to swiss cheese. Given that, it reminds me of the first crash I had in late '99. Although no one died, it was a horrible crash. When I saw the car a couple weeks later, I promptly threw up, if that gives you a reference point. A lady and I were sitting at a stop sign waiting to turn left on a busy road that passed over an interstate outside Indianapolis.

A kid came over the overpass from our left, was making a right on our street, and had no control. I remember him approaching the intersection, having his wheels turned right and sliding straight, and thinking "Dumb ass, get off your brakes!". When he didn't I leaned over, told the lady we were getting hit and tried shielding her.

That's my last memory for a few minutes. Overall, in the next four days I remember about 90 seconds total until waking up in a hospital bed with a morphine hangover, a caffeine headache and a throbbing in my abdomen like nothing I'd ever felt.

I remember trying to straighten, to help the EMT's pull me out of the car, them saying "Don't do anything, we'll do all the work", immobile, neck brace, darkness, rain on my face, I remember puking phlegm from my collapsed lungs into a tray in the emergency room, wondering if the nurse could read my expectorant like tea leaves…"Am I gonna live, sister?", darkness, tightly strapped on a gurney being wheeled across the roof to a waiting helicopter, rain in my face, loaded in and getting the attendants attention, her leaning over to me lifting the helmet from her ear to hear my astounding wisdom, to hear me whisper with my collapsed lungs "It's my first helicopter ride and you're not going to let me look out the fucking windows, are you?"and laughing, darkness, at University Medical in Indianapolis, the MRI or whatever humming and grinding to itself as light flashed across my eyelids, darkness, waking to see a woman with a straight razor zipping down my chest to remove the hair, thinking "Don't take my

133

fucking nipples off, lady." and then darkness....three days later.....alive.

     I woke up minus a spleen, but still alive. Ribs on my left side cracked just about all the way down. One lung that wouldn't reinflate for another two days until after they sent a camera/light/atomizer down my bronchial tube to remove a mucus clot. A staph infection that left me with a hernia that looked like I swallowed a basketball whole. But I was alive...

     Here's something for you. If you're in the last stages of treatment and reading this, you may need something to help you out, I've always thought this was funny.

     When I was in the hospital with this first wreck, my nurse partner told me walking was the best overall thing I could do. So from the time I was able, I dragged my ass outta bed every few hours, grabbed my IV tree and oxygen bottle, and took a short stroll. At first, it was out of bed, out the door, down the hall past the nurses station (sometimes just

134

to the nurses station), and back to my bed. By the last few days, it was laps around the floor after my second lung re-inflated.

So I set this goal in my mind, this certain day I was going to be out of there. I asked my nurses & doctors what I had to do to be out of there on my schedule, and one of the requirements was I had to have a bowel movement. Understand, by then I'd been 5 or 6 days on liquid nourishment, and hadn't taken a good solid crapper for almost a week.

So we get down to my D-day. I'm determined to be out of this hospital by sunset, and I had this *great* nurse that worked until about noon each day. The first time I saw her after she came on that day, I asked her how I could have a BM soonest. Now this is about 6AM, and she gave me these two little tiny pills. She said take those and it would help move things along.

About seven I had breakfast, my 3rd or 4th solid meal in a week, and around eight I had this incredible constant pain in my abdomen. Now, I've had gas before and the pain it can cause moving around, but that was nothing compared to this. I called the same nurse in and told her what was going on, could I have some medication for it? What I really told her was "I don't know what urban destruction bombs you gave me, but my gut feels like it's ready to explode." Anyway, she says "No, that's your bowel starting to work again…you did want to have a movement today, right?". Christ, I wanted to have a bowel movement, not a revolutionary-type social movement. Silly woman, it wasn't supposed to hurt like this!

Alright, I'm a creature of habit, I guess. Around 8 the same morning, I came swinging out my door with my IV tree (I had lost the oxygen tank by then) to take my walk. As you've probably figured out by now, I make some good connections wherever I'm at. Anyway, I walk by the nurse's station, and my nurse of the moment, the purveyor of gastric nightmares, leans over to another nurse and says loudly "Whatever you do, don't walk behind him today." and laughs her ass off!

Sad to say, she was completely right, once I started walking the gastric fireworks were in full swing. I may have killed the rest of the patients on the floor with my home-grown mustard gas during my walk, I don't know. I'm sure they were as glad as I was when my bowels moved and they could release me.

XXV

The reason I relate that is because the last 8 weeks of treatment, that's the closest comparison I can draw. I maintained from sunrise to sunset, I breathed in and out, I ate and I voided. The move from the big house to a smaller house is about all I remember clearly.

Please, please, don't let this scare you off. I had a great (comparatively) 18 weeks, but the last 8 weeks made up for it. You may experience this in your first weeks and learn how to deal with it, you may never experience this and wonder "What the hell is this wimp talking about?". It's okay either way, if you're dealing with what's going to kill you either way, understand?

One thing I do remember clearly is my last shots, especially the last four. I don't remember them individually, but collectively. Remember, tears are not one of my default emotions.

In the last few shots, leading up to it on Friday night I would sink deeper and deeper into what? Depression, resignation, I don't know what. Whatever it was, Friday afternoon it would start. By Friday at 9PM or so, I was not an emotional wreck, but an emotional black hole. Anything that came close to me I'd suck it in, and if it was positive I'd turn it to negative before integrating it. At 9PM, I'd turn into a diseased pumpkin, ready to return to the possessed castle, take my shot and die inside.

That was the most difficult part of treatment, Friday nights in the last six to eight weeks. My support lady was with me for every shot, and in the last four to six shots I really had to control my emotions. When I released that chemical poison into my leg and pulled the needle out, there were so many times when all I wanted to do was cry. I just wanted to submit to the emotional wreck and sob until it was over.

That wasn't an option, though. Given my personality, there was someone to shield from that, my support person of all people. There were also my kids, over alternating weekends, who couldn't see their dad in less that optimum condition. These were not conditions defined by my support lady or kids, understand that. These were *my* conditions, and weren't negotiable.

As a result, with fingernails and grit and intestinal fortitude I managed the last eight weeks. Whether you're in the first or the last eight weeks reading this, you can do it too. If you think you can't, call me. Email me. Smoke signals, eh? I don't care what, but get in touch with me. Call your nurses. Who is your support network?

XXVI

I thought I was doing well and fooling everyone close to me, but remember my support lady's daughter?

After treatment, my support and I were talking. During treatment my support lady, my kids, my quasi-kids, and my ex-s were all wonderful. Realistically, they all supported me when they could and where they could.

A. is one of my quasi-kids. I love her like my own daughter, she returns the favor, and there's not much more to say. Given that, after the move in mid-June, we didn't see a whole lot of her. Granted, she was busy with her life in Seattle, and she was 19, just busting out, all that stuff. But in talking with my support lady, I found out there was more to it than just that.

What I found out was that in the last eight weeks, which she hadn't been around for the majority of, she'd formed an opinion. The few times she'd seen me I hadn't "been myself". What she ended up telling her mom was she didn't want to come out just yet because she felt like I was dying, and she didn't want to be around for that.

Remember, this is when my nurse told my support they were taking a chest x-ray and if the results were off I was being admitted. This was when I just wanted to sob for the duration. This was when the thought of taking my next shot drove me into an emotional black hole....

I've seen her since getting off treatment, and it's much different. But just be aware, your emotions, your energy, your *chi*, all of that will be thrown off. If there are people in your life that are 'aware', they may distance themselves from you temporarily. Don't let it deter you. If you're going to do this, *do it!* Give them all the notice and information you can, they will support you as much as they can. But the bottom line is *just do it*. And there's people out here who will support you – your nurses, your staff, me, your support people, your family.

XXVII

Okay, we're on the homestretch now. Once I finished my treatments, I knew I had 6-12 months of recovery before I'd be anywhere close to 100%. My paperwork from August bears this out. Remember, this was taken about three weeks after treatment ended, and I'd started seeing some minor improvements.

However, I'm the type of person that feels 6-12 months only applies to humans. Superman wouldn't take a year to get back on top, so neither would I.

I see myself as a typical North American, carrying some extra weight, reasonably healthy and lazy, in the big picture. I know that Americans, myself included, walk probably less than 10% daily compared to other cultures.

A week and a day after my last shot, I knew I was on the road to recovery. I say that because after a week, my body was at the same spot it had been for the past 26 weeks. The next day was the first day in 26 weeks that the poison level in my system started to drop. This was exciting for me, to know the poisons in my body were starting to dissipate and flush out. That weekend was a kid weekend for me also, so it was a low key celebration for all of us, I think.

Saturday I went for a walk with the two youngest boys and my twin boys. We hadn't been on a hike for over a year, and while I wasn't trying to call this a hike I wanted to get out a bit and see how I handled it. Overall it went very well I thought.

We went to an area called Lord's Hill outside Snohomish that has miles of hiking trails without too much elevation gain or loss to deal with. We ended up hiking about 2.5-3 miles over an afternoon in a long loop. I found out what my limit was then, and

145

had a baseline to work from. By the end of the hike, muscles and joints were sore and stiffening, and I was ready for a nap!

We talked about drinking earlier, and what I'd do after treatment was over. I asked Pam what her thoughts were about two weeks before I took my last shot. She said she would think a beer or two a week wouldn't hurt, but to take it easy and monitor what the reactions were.

Once I got to where I was starting to mend, I tried a few beers. I started with one or two Red Stripes in the evening. Actually the first beer I tried was an Arrogant Bastard 22 oz., and that was a bit much, so I throttled back to something a little lighter that was still an independent brewery (I think). Besides, it's brewed in Jamaica, so it's probably healthy beer, right?

I got used to beer again, still loved it, and started drinking a bit too much on occasion. I felt alright, though, just had to stay aware of what my body was telling me. One thing that frustrated me was weight, which I'm sure alcohol isn't helping one bit.

During treatment I dropped about 20-25 pounds and a couple inches off my waist. That maintained for a couple months post-treatment, but then pants started getting tighter and that type of stuff.

My support lady had warned me that once off treatment I may rebound and actually be heavier if I wasn't careful. Well she was right, and so six months after treatment I have to look at changing my habits.

One of the things that I have to change is my activity level. During treatment I got into a sedentary routine simply because I didn't have energy to do otherwise. Now that treatment is over I realize the home-rest-work-home-rest routine that I'd gotten into has to change.

Here's something that blew my mind, one of my last epiphanies related to this treatment. As I'm sure you've recognized by now, I seem to think I'm a qualified amateur doctor, psychologist, dietician, naturopath, the list just goes on. This last realization came to me recently, after my final blood draw and test.

As we've discussed, I am also possibly an amateur alcoholic…and the amateur status is in doubt. Anyway, when I had my last appointment with the Girls, Kathleen told me I would have one final draw in about six months to make sure the virus didn't start reproducing again after the chemicals left my system. I was floored, because I was under the impression that with the six-month blood draw coming back negative and six months of chemicals in me, I was considered clean. This is where the 15-20% failure rate comes in.

Kathleen told me given my response to the treatment and the non-detection of the virus at this stage, she was reasonably confident it was gone. However, there was a chance it was dormant at a level they couldn't detect, and six months later would make that obvious if that was the case. You should understand, this virus is a sneaky bastard. Yes, it impacts the liver in a way that makes it detectable, but it incubates for 20 years sometimes before becoming active. In that time, it makes inroads in your liver, your bone marrow, effects your bodies ability to process protein, bile, carbohydrates, cholesterol, the list just goes on.

Well, suffice to say I was pissed, hacked, disappointed, scared, all of those and more, all in a quick second. Since I'd had to learn to keep my emotions under control during treatment, I managed to hang on for a minute and get things damped down.

I didn't realize how devastated I was until over six months after this news flash. But in retrospect, I see how I reacted and really need to share this with you, as you may find yourself in the same place, and hopefully this will help.

I drank lightly for probably 6 weeks after I'd taken the last shot. I liked where I was at then, 6 months dry and 6 weeks of seemingly being in control of my habits. But then things changed.

My drinking spiked to pre-treatment levels. Luckily, my moods and energy levels were still under control, as much as I had during this time. In hindsight, I think I recognize what was going on.

When treatment was done, I was supposed to be done, and finding out there was a chance it wasn't over switched something in my mind. Somewhere in there, I decided subconsciously that it wasn't over, that when I got re-tested I'd be positive again and looking at more treatment.

The Girls had told me it would be the same basic chemicals, but for 1-3 years this time depending on the viral load. I finally came to a decision 6 ½ months after treatment ended; if it would require more treatment, I wasn't doing it. I'd start my naturopathic regimen again that held it at bay, and I'd plan on doing that for the rest of my life. If it came down to treatment or nothing, I'd take the chances with that "nothing", but after being through treatment once, I never, ever, ever was willing to do it again.

About ten years ago, someone close to me asked me a question I answered truthfully. I knew it wasn't the answer they were expecting, but if someone asks me a direct question I feel obligated to give them a direct answer.

After their response, I started trying my best to live with a central standard. If I wanted to ask a question, I would first think of what would be the worst answer I could hear. This was my worst-case scenario. If I couldn't handle that answer, I wasn't ready to ask the question, simple as that.

In this case, my question was did I still have hep-c. The worst-case scenario I wasn't ready to accept, so I couldn't "ask" the question. Asking consisted of having my blood drawn and tested one last time.

So January came and went, and I didn't get tested. February got half done, and I hadn't been tested. But it weighed on me every day.

Finally I made the decision...I would get tested, but regardless of the results, I would not submit to the treatment again. If you're reading this before treatment, yes it is that bad. I don't want to scare you from taking the treatment if that's what you decide, but I want you to know that you can look back proudly after completion and say "Fuck you, I will *never* do this again!"

Here's the psychological part of this. I drank lightly, "responsibly", after treatment until that switch clicked over in my mind. Subconsciously I decided at that time, since I still had the virus in my scenario, that if anything was going to take me out it would be my choosing and my time. I knew that enough alcohol abuse would finish the job before the hep-c could, and my course was set.

This is amazing looking back on it. I had the blood drawn, printed a copy of this book, and went to see Pam at the clinic. We talked for a bit, and I asked her to proof this for me so if there were any glaring medical errors we could correct them.

I was at peace. I'd done the last test and decided on my course of action depending on the results. The craziest thing is when I gave blood, made up my mind and put the action behind it, my drinking throttled back substantially. The only explanation I have for it is that I was on the self-destruction path as long as I was living by my worst-case scenario.

A few days later I got a call early in the morning from a serious-sounding Pam. We gabbed for a bit about inconsequential things, but we both knew the real reason for the call. Finally Pam broke and told me I tested negative, no hepatitis-C virus detected after 6 months without medication. Levels of white and red blood cells were good, all other levels were good, and the biggest relief of all for me was that I still tested negative for pregnancy.

I'll give you this in closing…
schandler21@comcast.net

That email address has been mine for years, and I don't see it changing anytime soon. I won't be your doctor or nurse, but I'll help where I can.

You can do this. I won't sugar-coat anything and tell you it's easy, but it can be done, and on the other side, you'll look back and say "Yeah, it was bad, but it's over."

If it gets to be too much and you're wondering, drop me a line.

Things to remember:

1. With your nurses…communicate, communicate, communicate!
2. You may have symptoms treated by several doctors. Clinics differ, but my GI clinic was set up to treat the disease and monitor liver function, most other stuff I had to see my family doctor for. Don't let it get you down!
3. Choose your support person(s) carefully, they may be carrying you part of the way.
4. Prescriptions like anti-depressants and sleeping pills may be a necessary evil…but they may make the difference between completing or quitting.
5. It's frustrating, but symptoms and reactions are different for everyone. There's no consistency person to person, or even day to day…Take it a day at a time, and if you need to, take it minute by minute…you'll make it.

Notes:

It may help to note some of these names and
numbers early on...

Clinic: _____

Doctor: _____

Nurses: _____

_____

Support Network:

_____

_____

_____

_____

Steve Chandler, schandler21@comcast.net_____

Credits, and some general mopping up....

Cover Photo "Snohomish Sunrise" by Steve Chandler

Scuttlebutt logo and shirt reference used by permission of Scuttlebutt Brewing Co. Everett, WA...Thanks Young Phil and Old Phil!

Wedding photo by Elizabeth Tryon, used by permission...Thanks Brad and Karena, love you!

Editing and advice by Pam B...thank you so much!

About the author:

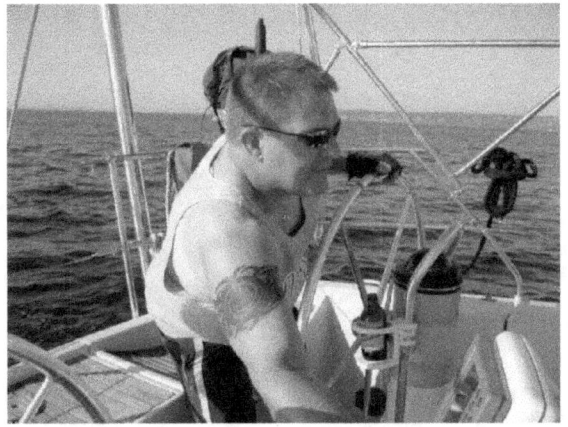

Steve currently lives in the Pacific NW with his family. This is his first book, but writing in the fantasy and adventure genres is in the works.

Additional copies can be ordered as printed or e-books at hepcman.com

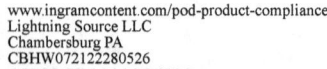